HEALTH
WITHOUT
DRUGS

Arabella Melville, Ph.D.
and
Colin Johnson

A Fireside Book
Published by Simon & Schuster Inc.
New York · London · Toronto · Sydney · Tokyo · Singapore

To our mothers,
Eva Johnson and Joan Melville,
who have retained some of the old wisdom.

And for the millions of animals who suffer
and die needlessly in the search for profitable drugs.

Fireside
Simon & Schuster Building
Rockefeller Center
1230 Avenue of the Americas
New York, New York 10020

Copyright © 1987 by Arabella Melville and Colin Johnson

All rights reserved
including the right of reproduction
in whole or in part in any form.

First Fireside Edition 1990
Published by arrangement with the authors

Originally published in Great Britain by Fontana Paperbacks.

FIRESIDE and colophon are registered trademarks
of Simon & Schuster Inc.

Designed by Irving Perkins Associates Inc.
Manufactured in the United States of America

3   5   7   9   10   8   6   4   2

Library of Congress Cataloging in Publication Data

Melville, Arabella.
Health without drugs / Arabella Melville and Colin Johnson.—1st
Fireside ed.
p.   cm.
"A Fireside book."
"Originally published in Great Britain by Fontana Paperbacks"—
T.p. verso.
Includes bibliographical references.
1. Self-care, Health.   2. Alternative medicine.   3. Drugs—Side
effects.   I. Johnson, Colin.   II. Title.
RA776.95.M45   1990
615.5—dc20   89-48725
                                                                          CIP
ISBN 0-671-68478-7

CONTENTS

	Foreword	9
	Introduction	12
	How to Use This Book	15
	PART 1: DRUGS IN PERSPECTIVE	17
1	Drugs and Health	19
2	Alternative Medicine	24
3	Everyday Drugs	30
	PART 2: CONDITIONS AND OPTIONS	39
4	Emotional Distress and Mental Illness	41
5	Colds and Respiratory Infections	66
6	Respiratory Allergies	82
7	Skin Disorders	102
8	Digestive Problems	115
9	Heart and Blood-Vessel Disease	133
10	Metabolic Problems	156
11	Liver, Kidneys and Bladder	171
12	Pain	189
13	Arthritis, Rheumatism and Joint Problems	214
14	The Reproductive System	225
15	Pregnancy and Birth	250

Contents

PART 3: HEALTH CHOICES   263

Introduction   265
16 Stress Management   266
17 Activity   283
18 Nutrition   296
19 How to Join the Healthy Minority   313

APPENDIXES   317

Appendix A: Information About Drugs and
  Health Care   319
Appendix B: Organic Food Suppliers   321
Appendix C: Bibliography   325
Index of Drug Names   329
General Index   334

FOREWORD

Since the end of World War II and the beginning of the modern "biomedical revolution," Western medicine has become increasingly dependent on pharmaceutical drugs and surgery as its treatments of choice for disease. It has become increasingly dependent on tests and technology for making its diagnoses. These developments have provided many benefits.

Routine surgery has become safer. New operations have been developed which have brought benefits in the treatment of certain kinds of cancer and heart disease, congenital defects and traumatic injury. Screening and early detection for several of the major killers has been significantly improved. The growth in the types and the use of the pharmaceutical drugs, the principal subject of this book, has provided many benefits—for example, in the management of diabetes, hypertension and certain infectious diseases. However, these advances and others have not been achieved without cost.

A significant number of unnecessary surgical operations are performed. Many unnecessary laboratory tests are carried out. And there is no known drug that is without side effects. Some of them are quite harmful, as this book makes clear. The excess surgery, lab testing and pharmaceutical drug use has thus produced unneeded discomfort, unnecessary disability and avoidable death.

In addition, during this era, health care costs in the United States have spiraled out of sight. In 1965 we spent $40 billion, approximately 6% of our gross national product (GNP), on health services. We are presently spending over $500 billion, 12% of our GNP, on health services. The United States spends a higher proportion of its GNP on health services than any other country in the world. (Not only do we spend huge sums on health services, but it is unclear just what benefits we have gained from this expenditure. Compared with

9

the other industrialized countries, we do not rank at the top on such health indicators as infant mortality rate and life expectancy. About 35 million of our people have no health insurance. And there are many serious deficiencies in the quality of medical care rendered.)

There are many factors accounting for this high level of expenditure. Among them is the increasing dependence on surgery, laboratory testing and sophisticated pharmaceutical drugs. More and more, medicine has been taken out of the home and the physician's office and put into the hospital. And hospitals are very expensive places in which to practice medicine. Our dependence on high-tech, hospital-based medicine is a major reason why our costs are so high. So pharmaceutical drugs cause health problems as well as solve them, and their extensive use contributes significantly to the rising costs of health care.

Furthermore, the focus on drugs and surgery, tests and technology, hospitals and inpatient care has increasingly made premature death the principal enemy of medicine. Modern Western medicine, with a few welcome exceptions, waits for people to get sick and then attempts to treat them, to return them to the state of being "not sick." Medicine's ultimate goal in persons who are seriously ill is nothing more, or less, than simply to cure disease and prevent premature death. But Western medicine tolerates the existence of disease.

Disease itself is not the principal enemy of Western medicine. If it were, there would be a major emphasis in our health-care delivery system on preventing people from getting sick in the first place. It is not as if we did not have a great deal of knowledge of how to prevent disease. We do. But it is simply not used. If we did use this knowledge, we could make disease rather than premature death the principal enemy, and premature death would become an increasingly rare event. Furthermore, we could significantly reduce the use of surgery, high-tech testing and pharmaceutical drugs.

Beyond prevention, in our "health" care delivery system there is little emphasis on health, which is much more than simply the absence of disease. Health can be defined as:

A state of well-being, of feeling good about oneself, of optimum functioning, of the absence of disease, and in which both internal and external risk factors are maximally controlled and/or reduced.

If health were to become the focus of medicine, as I believe it should, there would be even less need to use the pharmaceutical drugs.

In dealing with all of these issues, *Health Without Drugs* has three principal themes:

1. Pharmaceutical drugs inherently have the potential for harm, regardless of how great their potential benefit is.
2. If one does become ill, many alternative therapies other than drugs (or surgery), and preventive measures too, are available to help. These therapies can be both safe and effective if used correctly.
3. There are many ways to prevent illness and become healthy.

This book presents a detailed guide to virtually all of the major and many of the minor drugs in use today, both prescription and nonprescription. It briefly reviews how each of the body's major systems—cardiovascular, respiratory and so forth—works and what it does. The book describes the major illnesses of each system that can be treated with pharmaceutical drugs. It then describes the drugs that can be used, their benefits and their potential side effects.

Finally, it discusses various treatments and preventive alternatives available for dealing with the listed diseases, what the indications are for using those alternatives, what the evidence for their effectiveness is and what their risks are, if any. You will find that for many of them there are no potential deleterious side effects. At the very worst, there will simply be no benefit.

A constant theme of this book is the achievement and maintenance of health. Healthy living reduces the need to use pharmaceutical drugs. It is indeed the key to life. As Thomas Jefferson said, "Without health there is no happiness. An attention to health, then, should take the place of every other object." This book, used judiciously, will help you to avoid using pharmaceutical drugs when you don't need to, will help you to cure—without using drugs—sicknesses that may afflict you, and will help you to achieve a happy state of health.

—Steven Jonas, M.D.
Professor, Department of Community and Preventive Medicine
State University of New York at Stony Brook

INTRODUCTION

The alternative which this book offers is the creation of health in place of illness. Advocates of "alternative" as opposed to conventional pills will for the most part not find what they seek in the recommendations we make. No matter what your current condition, the strategies we offer for dealing with specific illnesses are designed to improve your health rather than to cosset your disease or suppress your symptoms.

In recent years people have become wary of swallowing the pills that many doctors automatically prescribe at consultations. Thirty years ago there was universal acceptance of drug treatment; after the miracle of penicillin we entered the age of "a pill for every ill," when only cranks questioned the good that ever-increasing quantities of drugs would bring. Then came thalidomide and a rude awakening.

Slowly it became apparent that throwing drugs at every symptom or problem was not a rational way to treat illness. Worse, research showed that drug therapy, far from creating health, was in fact creating illness. Iatrogenic disease—literally, doctor-caused disease, but usually taken to mean illness caused by side effects of drugs or adverse reactions to them—became a widespread addition to the disease load in every country.

After thalidomide, governments made much of controlling the excesses of drug manufacturers and ensuring that adverse drug reactions were monitored. This had little effect; as we documented in our book *Cured to Death: The Effects of Prescription Drugs*, major drug tragedies continued to kill or maim thousands. We concluded that prescription drugs cause roughly the same number of casualties each year as road accidents. Despite many differences between countries, in controls and attitudes to medicine, this rule of thumb holds good wherever health professions have been seduced by the idea that drugs offer quick and easy answers.

Most people now accept that there is no such thing as a safe drug. Most of us are prepared to tolerate a degree of risk in certain circumstances in return for the possibility of benefits—the risk/benefit ratio—yet doctors and drug manufacturers generally remain either ignorant or unrealistic about risk while talking enthusiastically and equally unrealistically about benefit. The truth is that many of them simply assume without question that modern drug therapy is beneficial.

Drugs are rarely rigorously tested to prove their benefits under the conditions in which they are actually used, so there is a lack of objective sources of information for consumers on hazards and risk/benefit ratios. This, along with the increasing breakdown of trust in doctors, has led to the wariness many feel about swallowing their medicine.

Behind this wariness is a growing realization that drugs do not produce the health that was promised, that our reliance upon them has been misplaced, that we have in some very basic way been misled. Perhaps we should not be surprised at this. We have asked doctors to treat illness, not to create health. In asking the wrong question we have been led into a cul-de-sac. By treating symptoms, or even diseases, we do not create health; at best we buy time, during which we should instead address the question of the *causes* of illness. We have failed to understand that human health is *not* the same as the absence of symptoms, illness or disease.

The preconditions for a positive state of health, in which we may each fulfill our potential, are beginning to be understood and defined. The information given in this book, although in many ways simple, is at the frontiers of this new understanding. It is based upon a holistic view of humans as composite beings in which mind, body and spirit are integrated and which live within a biosphere which is itself a dynamic and interacting composite of many life forms. At its widest, holism states that the health of the person is dependent on the health of the planet; you cannot expect to be healthy in an unhealthy world.

The holistic approach does not exclude any possibilities in its search for health. It is a philosophy which allows you to have your cake and eat it too—provided that you keep the question of cake in perspective. So while the alternatives to drugs suggested in this book are designed to alleviate symptoms and remove conditions, there will be occasions when we say, "Take the drugs." There are circumstances and conditions for which there are no alternatives to drugs, and others for which they provide the best if not the only answer.

We are therefore not dogmatically antidrug. Indeed, to be so would be fatally irrational for one of us (an insulin-dependent diabetic). Our position is this: drugs are useful in many circumstances where there is no safer alternative and where their potential risks and benefits are understood. If these two preconditions of use were generally accepted, the consumption of drugs would drop by around 90% and most of the death and disaster associated with their profligate misuse would disappear.

The overwhelming advantage of the alternatives to drugs which we suggest is that they *will* create health. Starting from the condition which may be troubling you, the strategies we offer will allow you to deal with the immediate problem, give you some insight into the cause, and then encourage you to go on to make simple adjustments in your life which will allow you to experience health rather than disease. This is something no drug will ever do.

Arabella Melville
Colin Johnson
Lowestoft
Suffolk
England

H O W   T O   U S E
T H I S   B O O K

This book is designed to be used as a reference source. Few people will want to read about all the illnesses and conditions covered, so the following suggestions are intended to help you get the best use of it, whatever your particular interest.

First, if you wish to get some general idea of current drug usage and problems, and the place of alternative medicine in treating sickness, read part 1.

Next, with a notebook ready, consult the relevant sections of part 2 for your condition. Some of these may overlap, such as digestive and metabolic disorders, so you may find yourself reading more than one section to cover a particular condition. Use the introductory paragraphs and the section index which follows them to make sure you are on the right track.

The drugs used to treat your condition will be listed along with their serious side effects and common adverse reactions. If you are taking tablets or other medicines but do not know precisely what for, look them up in the drug glossary and you will be referred to the relevant section. Drugs may be prescribed which are normally used for another condition—e.g., cough mixture for insomnia. In this type of case, the drug will be in the list relevant to the condition for which it is normally used. So readers will need to refer to the glossary.

When reading about your condition you will find references to other sections in the book (for example, "see section 17.2," or "see section 18.4(b)"). Make a note of these as you go. When you have collected all the references relevant to your condition, go on to part 3.

The introductory section of each chapter in part 3 explains general principles. Read these before going on to the specific references which you have noted when reading about your problem. Then, when working through the recommendations, note the actions you have to take to implement them, such as changing your grocery list, getting time for relaxation and so on.

Finally, at the end of the book are listed various organizations which can help you or which you can join to help others, and details on books for further reading.

PART 1

DRUGS
IN
PERSPECTIVE

1

Drugs and Health

AMERICA is a nation of drug takers. Every day, the majority of Americans will use tablets, potions, suppositories, creams or lotions containing one or more drugs. In 1986, the average U.S. citizen spent $122 on six prescriptions; year by year, the drug bill rises. Americans have become so accustomed to using drugs whenever a health problem arises that it is accepted as quite rational to use them on a daily basis just to maintain normality and cope with everyday life.

Why should this be cause for concern? Basically because medicines cannot produce good health. All too often, they contribute to the problem of illness, adding the extra burden of drug-induced disease.

There is no such thing as a safe drug. Every substance which has a pharmacological effect may also have side effects and be capable of producing a whole range of potentially serious adverse effects. Side effects are effects other than those intended; for example, an antihistamine taken for hay fever, a cold or travel sickness may also cause drowsiness. Side effects are not necessarily harmful in themselves, although they may set off a range of dangerous secondary effects. Drowsiness may be no problem if you're a passenger in a car, but if you're driving, your use of an antihistamine could put others at risk. Adverse reactions are more serious. They range from skin rashes and nausea to permanent disruption of the body's metabolic systems and death. Even the safest drugs, like penicillin, kill hundreds of people in the United States every year.

The problem with unwanted drug effects is that they often seem unpredictable. And they depend on the individual who takes the drug as much as on the drug itself. So while one person may be fine on a particular drug, someone else could become very ill from it. No matter how carefully drugs are tested, it is only through many years of use by thousands of people that some of the problems they can cause are discovered. Unfortunately, by then it is too late for many of the victims.

Drug-induced illness is very common. It has been estimated that there are between 5 and 10 million adverse drug reactions in the United States every year. Unfortunately, there are no precise figures because there is no reliable information. The FDA is informed of about 12,000 adverse drug reactions each year, but this is no guide to the actual number because most drug-induced illness is never reported. Usually, it is just treated as a new condition; the unfortunate victim is given more drugs and thus exposed to even greater risk.

This is not the result of carelessness, ignorance, or malice. It is a predictable effect of the nature of Western medicine and our cultural assumptions, combined with the uncertainty of diagnosis. For example, beta blockers, commonly used for heart conditions and increasingly for anxiety, can cause diabetes. But it is almost impossible to distinguish between drug-induced diabetes and diabetes which may develop in people who have never taken beta blockers, so it is very unlikely that the diabetes will be recognized as an adverse drug reaction.

Adverse reactions to therapy can be both unpredictable and unavoidable; whenever drugs are used, adverse reactions will sometimes occur. Even adverse reactions that could have been predicted and should be recognized are unlikely to be correctly diagnosed. The doctor may fear the possibility of a malpractice suit, and no doctor wants to believe that his actions have caused harm; so he will naturally tend to prefer another explanation for the illness. Research projects designed to detect adverse drug reactions discover rates that are much higher than most doctors acknowledge; a typical finding of American hospital-based research is that one patient in five suffers from drug-induced illness.

When we take medicines, we cannot be sure what their effects are going to be. We hope for benefit but we may be damaged; we hope that the drugs will be effective but cannot know until we have taken the risk. We take drugs on trust, hoping that the prescribing doctor has judged correctly and that we will not be the ones to suffer. Our trust is based on faith in doctors and in the government controls on drug availability. Is such trust justified?

Regrettably, to rely on doctors' understanding of the actions of drugs is to put ourselves in the hands of a shockingly poorly educated and misinformed group. Medical courses may take many arduous years, but very little of that time is devoted to pharmacology, the study of drugs. Until recently, many medical schools taught no pharmacology at all. Even now, pharmacology represents a trivial part of most medical school courses. What knowledge doctors may have acquired in training is often out of date by the time they come to apply it. New products, not necessarily more effective, safer or even needed, come onto the market at an alarming rate as the drug manufacturers strive to maintain their enviable profit records. So doctors actually have a very limited theoretical understanding of their most frequently used therapeutic approach. They take drugs on trust, just as their patients do.

The main source of information about drugs for both doctors and patients is the pharmaceutical industry which produces and markets medicines. It is in the best interest of these companies to keep the use of their products as high as possible; as one graffiti artist at a famous Northeastern medical school put it, "The makers of aspirin wish you had a headache right now!" Drug corporations are not philanthropic bodies; they are among the most powerful and profitable businesses in the world.

Naturally, the companies work at selling their products by emphasizing benefits and playing down hazards. And their message is put over so strongly and effectively that many doctors neither acknowledge the dangers of drug therapy nor offer any other way of dealing with common forms of illness.

While doctors put their faith in the drug companies for information about drugs, it is the government's task to protect the public from the potential excesses of the pharmaceutical industry. The FDA's Bureau of Drugs is the most sophisticated body of its kind in the world; it assesses new drugs, monitors established drugs in use, controls advertising and polices the industry. However, its effectiveness is hampered by political priorities and the long legal battles that ensue when it attempts to control profitable products.

Unlike its counterparts in countries such as Norway, the FDA is not permitted to base its judgments on questions of need for drugs; all it can ask is that a new product be proved safe and effective. Even this is difficult when some laboratories and investigators regularly produce false or misleading data.

Nevertheless, the FDA has succeeded in protecting Americans from some of the worst drug disasters experienced in Europe. Thalidomide, responsible for thousands of malformed babies, was never permitted in the United States; nor was Eraldin, a heart drug that maimed thousands in Britain in the mid-1970s. Many of the more dubious preparations available in Britain and Europe are not available in the United States. Regrettably, the FDA cannot control the export activities of American drug companies; drugs judged too dangerous for the American people are sold abroad, where drug regulation is less effective.

No matter how good drug regulation may be, however, the underlying problems with medicines remain. Drugs are rarely capable of *curing* illness; what they do is control the symptoms, leaving the cause untouched. Perhaps as much as 90% of primary-care consultations are for conditions which medicine cannot cure—conditions which result from unsatisfactory relationships, poor diet or housing, lack of knowledge or understanding. Yet the majority of those who consult a doctor will receive a prescription for products which, while they might make them feel a little better, will certainly not restore them to wellness.

Research has shown that the main determinant of what the doctor prescribes, and whether he prescribes at all, is not the patient's condition but the doctor's own attitudes. His advice is as likely to be based on prejudice as knowledge. Doctors everywhere have developed habits of unnecessary, inappropriate or frankly dangerous prescribing—and patients are suffering.

This situation has developed because we have been seduced by the powerful idea of a "magic bullet." The idea was developed by a German chemist, Paul Ehrlich, around the beginning of this century. The magic bullet of Ehrlich's imagination was capable of seeking out and killing parasites in the body without harming the host in any way. But the magic bullet proved illusory. No drug acts in this way; all are capable of causing harm. Yet Western doctors continue to practice medicine as though drugs were entirely benign.

There can be no doubt that in many cases medicine does succeed. Millions owe their lives to the timely use of antibiotics, to routine vaccination or replacement therapy. Many who suffer from pain or metabolic disorders find relief which may be achieved in no other way. But while drugs *can* be good and appropriate, their overuse is not.

Paradoxically, minimum use of drugs confers maximum benefit. Medicine should be the last resort, not the first. If illness can be resolved by natural means, through an appropriately balanced lifestyle and other risk-free measures, the benefits will be greater than can be achieved through the use of any medicine. Risk should never be underestimated or dismissed; it must be considered, and the safest methods should be tried before we turn to the less safe.

Instead of regarding symptoms as things to get rid of, we need to take heed of their meaning, trying to understand what imbalances exist in our lives so that we may remedy them and thus become symptom-free. To suppress symptoms indiscriminately with drugs is like switching off your alarm systems; such warnings should be heeded, not suppressed. When we change our attitudes in this way, we shall be creating health rather than servicing an ever-increasing level of illness.

2

Alternative Medicine

IN recent years there has been a boom in what is loosely termed "alternative" or "complementary" medicine. This has been stimulated by a growing awareness of the conventional drug cul-de-sac described in the previous chapter, and by a reaction against the impersonal nature of treatment offered by the conventional health services.

The important point about alternative medicine is that although it may use different techniques, or have originated in other cultures, it is still aimed at treating illness, not at creating health. Some alternative systems are based on the concept of the *restoration* of health, but in our culture it is doubtful whether they in fact achieve this. In absorbing these techniques we have inevitably changed them; they are all now characterized by the passive nonparticipation of the patient in relation to the expert (healer, masseur, operator or doctor) which is typical of conventional medicine.

The outstanding advantage offered by many alternatives to conventional medicine is that they are far less dangerous. While they may or may not be considered effective, they rarely harm those who use them. This undoubtedly contributes to their popularity with patients.

The best-established alternative system is *homeopathy*. It is used by the British royal family and has practitioners in most parts of the country. Homeopathy uses like to cure like—very dilute solutions of substances which in higher doses induce the symptoms from which the patient suffers. The precise way in which these microdoses work is not known, but they seem to give the body a chance to make a subtle assessment of the substance and act appropriately.

The substances involved vary widely. They include a vast range of herbs and plant products, infectious organisms derived from the things which cause illness, and minerals such as sulphur. Whereas in conventional medicine a higher dose of a drug is given to achieve a greater effect, in homeopathy the opposite is the case. The more homeopathic medicines are diluted the more powerful they are deemed to be; a homeopath would be quite happy for you to have a lump of sulphur in your possession but he would be concerned if you had sugar pills made from a dilution of sulphur so great that none of the original molecules could, in theory, be present. Despite the apparent illogicality of this there is accumulating scientific evidence that such preparations do have biological effects.

Homeopathic remedies have to be chosen with care. A sympathetic consultation with a homeopath will provide an insight into your life-style that will enable him or her to correct your symptoms and make suggestions for changes which will prevent their recurrence. Self-treatment with over-the-counter remedies is often ineffective, but the skilled application of carefully selected remedies can produce spectacular results. Allergic and autoimmune conditions seem to respond particularly well.

Unfortunately, homeopathy has become tainted with the conventional medical approach. Some practitioners fail to assess their patients with care—taking regard of all their personal qualities as well as the nature of their symptoms—but instead merely dish out prescriptions as a conventional doctor might. Their remedies are not likely to do any harm, but under these circumstances they are not likely to do much good either.

Osteopaths and *chiropractors* depend upon manipulation of the body to realign bones and joints. Their treatments are not always risk-free, but the risks are very low with experienced practitioners. Osteopathy has recently been found acceptable by the medical establishment, although it still tends to be kept at arm's length. Some practitioners work in much the same way as physiotherapists, focusing on particular parts of the body, manipulating, sometimes applying liniments, heat and/or cold. Others claim to be able to sort out a wide range of problems by manipulation alone. As with most systems of medicine, the claims of some practitioners are undoubtedly exaggerated, but in many cases their methods produce remarkable results. They have a reputation for being particularly good for back pain.

Acupuncture involves the stimulation of specific points of the body by fine needles in order to excite or block a reaction in connected body systems. The most spectacular use of acupuncture is practiced by the Chinese to block pain for surgery. Modern substitutes for fine needles, which incidentally do not usually hurt, include electrical stimulation, heat, and finger pressure on the acupuncture points. The finger-pressure technique can be useful for dealing with pain such as earache. Acupuncture is used for treating a wide range of problems, from chronic pain to metabolic disorders, although the range of treatments offered will vary from practitioner to practitioner.

The Chinese doctors who developed acupuncture saw it as a way of rebalancing the whole body and thus conferring health; Western practitioners today tend to view it as a way of reducing unpleasant symptoms. The advantage of acupuncture is that it does not in any way damage the patient provided that the needles are sterile, but it does not work for everyone, nor will it permanently reverse the effects of living in ways which induce illness.

Herbal remedies are found in all cultures, and they are the foundation upon which modern drug therapy is built. Some of the remedies in wide use have been tested by modern medicine and incorporated as part of its pharmacopoeia. Aspirin, derived originally from the bark of the willow tree, is one example. Digitalis, which comes from the foxglove and is used for heart disease, is another.

A common misconception about herbal remedies is that they are safer than modern drugs; because they are natural they are thought to be in some way benign. In fact herbs can be quite as dangerous as any synthetic medicine. The general rule for herbs is exactly the same as that for conventional medicines: the more potent their properties, the more dangerous they are likely to be.

Taking herbal remedies for illness is therefore basically no different from taking drugs from the chemist. The medicines may come from natural sources, but the underlying idea and the types of effects to be expected are much the same. However, just as you are not likely to suffer serious damage from an over-the-counter product bought from a pharmacist, so you will probably come to no harm with feverfew from your garden or the herbal mixture you buy at your local health store. Nevertheless herbalists, like doctors, should have extensive knowledge of the substances they prescribe. The wonderful old lady down the road can no more be relied upon because she deals in herbs than can her neighbor who believes her latest medicine to be the most fantastic cure-all; so caution is advisable if you are considering using herbs for any problem, and you should go to a well-established and reputable practitioner.

Herbalists vary in their approaches. Some tend, like conventional doctors, to focus on symptoms and prescribe specific remedies for them; others, in accordance with a holistic tradition, will endeavor to consider the whole person and discuss many aspects of life-style. A good herbalist can be a valuable guide both to herbal medicines and to eating and activity patterns that will help you.

Orthomolecular medicine is the most recent development in this field. In one sense it is an alternative approach, since it attempts to rebalance the body, but at the same time it shares the narrow "scientific" approach of modern medicine. This method uses large doses of vitamins and minerals, sometimes in conjunction with drug therapy, to deal with illness. While some of the successes claimed by orthomolecular practitioners are spectacular, large quantities of specific nutrients must be used with great care because, like drugs, they can produce serious adverse effects. *Never attempt to treat yourself with megadoses of vitamins or minerals;* you are not likely to solve your problems in this way and you could find yourself suffering a new set of symptoms.

Faith healers have the longest tradition of all, and they are also enjoying a current vogue. Their methods are quite different from those of the other healers described in this chapter, and indeed are largely dismissed by both alternative and conventional medical practitioners. Faith healers do achieve results which, if inexplicable, are nonetheless real. In our culture, healers tend to be motivated by Christian beliefs aided by a belief in contact with agencies beyond themselves.

Healers work by focusing attention and energy on their relaxed subjects. Without prior knowledge they can locate problem areas of the body. Subjects report heating of those parts the healer is focusing upon; increased movement in stiffened joints is common, as is the subsidence of pain. The healer may or may not touch the subject, yet the results are much the same. There have been no studies of the long-term efficacy of such treatment, but there are records of remarkable successes. While we can offer no explanation for it, we nevertheless believe that it cannot be dismissed. It certainly does no harm, and the relaxation necessary in the subject is totally beneficial.

All these alternative options are frequently described as *holistic,* a term which in medical usage implies that the person is treated as a whole integrated being, a compound of mind, body and spirit. It is used to differentiate alternative systems from the mechanistic approach of conventional medicine, which treats the human body as a series of electrochemical events summarized in physical action. The mechanistic view of health leads to the impersonal approach of doctors who treat people as a collection of symptoms to be modified in isolation. Holism is much wider than this; it is essentially a philosophy which includes everything and seeks to give it perspective. Thus holists believe that the health of the person is inseparable from the health of the planet and all its life, and that any cure which does not educate the sufferer in the widest parameters of his or her condition is nonsense.

Whatever system you try for relief of illness, you should not lose sight of the fact that the need for any treatment at all is a symptom of failure in basic health maintenance. The need to correct basics in order to achieve health is our reason for adopting a holistic perspective of human existence. Without this you will continually have to resort to one or another type of curative approach. Cures are limited; they work for a while until the disease (or another form of disease) reasserts itself in the imbalanced person. As a society we waste untold time, money and energy trying to treat disease rather than to prevent it. The irrationality of this approach is illustrated by cancer: it is reliably estimated that 80% of the cancers we suffer are environmental in origin and are therefore avoidable, yet we rarely address the question of the causes of cancers, preferring to pursue the illusion of cure.

While alternative systems clearly share many of the characteristics of conventional medicine, they tend to be safer. We would therefore recommend that you explore what they have to offer if you need help with an intractable problem. Different methods tend to vary in their efficacy according to the condition and individual involved, but if you can find one that works for you it will be better than the conventional answer of suppressing symptoms with drugs.

3

Everyday Drugs

WHEN we consider everyday drugs, the question of perspective becomes paramount. In the Christian West alcohol is a sacrament, but in the Islamic East it is abhorred. Every culture has its own drugs for recreation, celebration and stimulation, and because of the way we are all conditioned within our culture we view the practices of other cultures as unnatural, dangerous or downright evil. But in spite of these differences of opinion there are very few humans who take no drugs at all.

It is important when considering questions of health to understand the effects these substances may have on us, for although they may be regarded as "normal," "acceptable" or legal within our society their status usually has little or nothing to do with their effects on the health either of individuals or of society as a whole.

First let us define exactly what we mean by a drug. A drug is *any substance which alters the state of mind or body beyond that which would normally occur.* The most prevalent drugs are those with which we are all familiar: nicotine in tobacco, alcohol in a wide range of drinks, caffeine and its close relatives such as theobromine in coffee, tea, cocoa and cola drinks. All the substances we use as medicines are drugs, whether prescribed or bought over the counter. The media keep before us the problems with illegal or "street" drugs such as heroin, cocaine, crack, marijuana and so on, though drug abuse is probably more common with prescribed drugs, and many of the same substances are used by both medical patients and junkies.

These drugs form a hierarchy or pyramid of perceived danger. Heroin has been at the top for some time, but is now threatened by crack, a cocaine derivative which can be smoked and is said to be instantly addictive. Below this come the other street drugs, and these overlap with the more commonly abused prescription drugs such as barbiturates, amphetamines and tranquilizers. Nicotine heads the list of dangerous everyday drugs, followed by alcohol, with caffeine and other mild ubiquitous stimulants forming the base of the pyramid. We would stress that this hierarchy is only loosely related to the *actual* harm caused by the drugs; questions such as religion, politics, taxability, habit and custom are very influential.

The usual problem associated with drug use is that of addiction. There are two extreme forms of drug addiction: the first is usually associated with narcotics such as opium and its derivatives, which induce sleepiness or euphoria and change the addict's metabolism so that bodily systems are reluctant to function in the absence of the drug; the second is caused by drugs such as tranquilizers which alter consciousness and perception in such a way that the addicts become anxious without the drug and feel they cannot cope, or can cope better if they have it. Many drugs work at both physical and psychological levels, the balance depending on the individual, which makes dealing with addiction far from straightforward. The simple truth about addiction is that *any* drug can become addictive. Not all people who use heroin become addicted, while millions feel very deprived without their regular cup of coffee.

Below our pyramid of street, prescribed and everyday drugs there are many other substances, such as sugar, which are addictive but are not considered to be drugs at all. Sugar and artificial sweeteners give us an energy rush. They also cause an insulin overrun which makes our blood sugar drop. We then have to eat more food or take more sugar. Because we are programmed to eat sweet things—in nature these would be seasonal fruits—manufacturers of everything from slimming foods to baked beans add sugar to their products. For the manufacturers there are two benefits: it increases sales and it helps preserve the product. For the consumer the effects are far from beneficial: a large part of the illnesses and ailments suffered in the United States can be attributed to our addiction to sugar.

Salt—more correctly, sodium salts in their many forms—is also addictive. One effect of oversalted food is a slow rise in blood pressure. Increased blood pressure is a part of the body's natural response to stress or injury, helping to cushion us both physically and psychologically against trauma. Our bodies quickly learn this, and we find ourselves reaching for the salt even before we have tasted the food. Manufacturers have also learned this, and they put salt in almost everything, alongside the sugar and for exactly the same reasons.

Other substances in food, such as additives and a wide range of drug and pesticide residues, are treated by our bodies as toxins. Toxic stress causes a small surge of adrenaline when we eat foods containing these substances. If we regularly consume food and drink contaminated by them we can become addicted to the adrenaline surge they produce.

The problem of everyday drugs is therefore a wide one. The effects on health are difficult to quantify because of the different reactions they produce in different people. Despite evidence that a significant number of people are adversely affected by some additives, all the additives put into processed food are considered safe by the authorities and the food industry, and they have held hands and fought a rearguard action against increasing public concern. In this respect they are very similar to the government and drug industry alliance, which comes as little surprise when you learn that drug manufacturers are often the same companies that make the veterinary drugs which contaminate meat, the pesticides which contaminate land and crops, and the vast range of chemicals used both as additives and processing intermediaries in the food industry. The food they present to us as normal, desirable and convenient must therefore be looked at with deep suspicion if we are concerned about our health and that of our families. (Fuller discussion of this subject can be found in Chapter 18, where advice is given on eating well and safely.)

For most people stimulants are the order of the day, whether taken as a cup of tea in bed, or coffee with the cornflakes, or that mug of hot chocolate at night. *Theobromine* and *theophylline,* caffeinelike drugs found in tea and chocolate, are mildly addictive stimulants. *Caffeine* is found in coffee, tea, cocoa and colas. It is also used in many over-the-counter tonics, pick-me-ups and pain relievers. Caffeine is a stimulant which aids alertness and wakefulness. Addicts, drinking five or more cups of strong coffee a day, are liable to develop stress-related diseases. Whether this is directly caused by caffeine consumption, or by the circumstances that lead the person to become dependent on the drug in the first place, is unclear. Caffeine-sensitive people often suffer from insomnia if they get into the habit of drinking coffee in the evening.

A side effect of tea and coffee is that they act as diuretics, making the body lose water. Many tea drinkers who *retain* excessive water may be doing so as a reaction to this imposed shedding. If they are then prescribed more diuretics the problem can get worse and complications with blood pressure follow.

Nicotine is one of the most dangerous drugs in widespread use today. Cigarette smoking has been identified as the chief avoidable cause of death in the United States. According to the Centers for Disease Control, 15.7% of all U.S. mortality in 1984—a total of 320,515 deaths—was attributable to smoking. Over the past few decades, three separate presidential commissions have recommended an outright ban on tobacco on health grounds. Unfortunately, because of the numbers of addicts and the tax revenue they produce, no government has felt able to take this logical step. Cigarette smokers put themselves and others at risk of lung cancer and heart and circulatory disease. Smoking also increases the risk of cancers of the liver, pancreas and cervix. Dealing with these conditions, and amputating legs damaged by the effects of smoking on blood vessels, bleeds away time and resources from health care in every country in the world. As enlightenment spreads in the West and more people give up smoking, cigarette companies increase their export efforts to the Third World, where health education is practically nonexistent. The results will be entirely predictable and, like most drug dealing, very profitable.

The physical effects of nicotine which keep addicts hooked and make it so difficult to stop smoking are quite remarkable. Nicotine is the only drug which is both stimulant and tranquilizer. It aids alertness while calming anxiety and reducing boredom. It is undoubtedly a very potent drug, which is why so many people are addicted to smoking every bit as badly as heroin addicts are to their fix.

Alcohol is another killer, although it has some mitigating features. Alcohol is believed to kill between one and two hundred thousand people in the United States annually. And as we drink more each year, more people succumb to the direct effects of long-term alcohol poisoning, cirrhosis and cancers of the liver. Alcohol also has undesirable secondary effects in the body, causing dehydration through overstimulation of the kidneys and interfering with the absorption of vitamins from food. Metabolizing alcohol can put severe strain on the liver, and hangovers result when the liver is temporarily overloaded with alcohol and the other toxic substances which are present in drinks.

Alcohol is a disinhibitor. It reduces the strength of the mental forces which restrain us on our particular straight and narrow. One of the inhibiting forces is anxiety; alcohol gives us a little confidence, makes us think we are doing better than we actually are, or stops us worrying about how or what we are doing. Although we may not realize it at the time, our judgment is actually impaired and the precision of our movements is disrupted. This is why it causes road accidents. Alcohol can also release aggressive or sexual behavior by reducing the social inhibitions which normally control such impulses. On the whole alcohol, although its use is universally accepted and encouraged, is far more harmful than marijuana, the use of which is prohibited.

Despite the real dangers of excessive alcohol use, moderate consumption (provided you are not an alcoholic, for whom *any* amount of alcohol means trouble) does not seem to do any harm. In fact people who drink a little, on average one drink per day, actually live longer than those who avoid alcohol altogether. Whether this is an effect of the alcohol or the effect of the social contact often involved in drinking is not known.

Over-the-counter drugs (OTCs) are medicines that are considered relatively free from adverse effects. They can be bought in any quantity for any use. Those considered more hazardous are restricted to sale in pharmacies. All OTC medicines in fact carry some risk, and can also be addictive, as was illustrated some years ago in Glasgow when many people were found to be taking Askit Powders, a preparation mainly consisting of aspirin, in the belief that it prevented colds. It did not, and the excessive consumption was discovered because of the high incidence in the area of stomach ulcers and intestinal bleeding.

Illicit drugs, or drugs which are used illicitly, are seen as a cause for growing concern as greater numbers of young people become addicted to certain street drugs. Whether it is the addiction per se which troubles the authorities (who are after all happy to take the revenue from tobacco sales), or the secondary social problems such as petty crime, violence, prostitution, disruption of education or discontinuity of social values which accompany addiction, is a matter of debate. In many parts of the world authorities are content to allow, if not encourage, drug use as a means of damping down wider social unrest. The thriving colony of Hong Kong with its exemplary business ethic was originally built on the British government-backed opium trade.

The question of abusing *solvents* is not quite in the mainstream of drug abuse. The many volatile substances in everyday use are so highly poisonous that their use must more properly be regarded as a method of committing suicide. These substances produce illusions and a sense of floating and timelessness, followed by nausea, slurred speech and confusion. Ulcers appear on the nose and mouth; liver, kidney and lung damage follow, and blood disorders, gastroenteritis and sometimes heart failure can occur.

The mainstream illicit drugs do not form a homogeneous group. The reasons for declaring a drug illegal are largely subjective, and there is usually much hypocrisy in the application of the law to users. For many years cocaine was a smart jet-set drug, attracting few prosecutions among users, while marijuana was pursued among ethnic groups with comparative vigor, resulting in draconian prison sentences.

Cannabis or *marijuana* (also known as grass, ganja, weed, pot and

other names which reflect the origin or nature of the particular form)
is a drug which is very widely used by people in all social groups in
America and in most other countries of the world. Its use in some
countries has been decriminalized. Cannabis can produce relaxation, lethargy, incoordination, loss of motivation and euphoria. It
can also intensify moods, produce heightened sensitivity to a wide
range of stimuli, disturb short-term memory and promote free-
flowing ideas and strange fantasies. Its main adverse effects are panic
and nausea, especially when used with tobacco.

There seem to be few, if any, long-term hazards associated with
cannabis use. Until the early years of this century it was used for pain
relief—Queen Victoria used tincture of cannabis for menstrual
pains—and it is used today in cancer treatment. While interference
with memory may reflect changes in the brain, the fact that the
powerful anticannabis lobby has been unable to document serious
damage to any body system indicates that the dangers to individual
health must be minor. Habituation to cannabis occurs with regular
use, and deprivation can lead a heavy user to become depressed and
edgy.

LSD (d-lysergic acid diethylamide, or "acid"), the psychedelic
drug of the sixties, produces intense effects on the mind and very
little effect on the body. It is one of the most potent drugs known to
man; doses are measured in micrograms, and a minute quantity can
have incredible impact. Its effects vary widely with the mood and
personality of users, their expectations and the circumstances sur-
rounding the "trip." In general it increases the speed of mental
activity, and causes perceptual and visual distortion. Hallucinations
are common. Users can suffer extreme panic, fear and depression—
the "bad trip"—or they may enjoy a sense of joy and peace, feelings
of insight and deeply religious, spiritual or mystical experiences. LSD
can trigger lasting mental breakdown in susceptible people, and
recovery can take several months. Users have reported dropping
back into trips weeks or months after the drug-induced experience
occurred—a particularly worrying phenomenon among people
whose normal occupation is flying bombers or patrolling in nuclear
submarines. Addiction to LSD is unlikely because the drug ceases to
have any effect if it is taken frequently, and larger doses do not

overcome this block. Paradoxically, experienced users often require smaller doses of the drug.

Cocaine and *amphetamine* are stimulant drugs. They are often mixed, or "cut," because amphetamine is much cheaper than cocaine and the two have similar effects. These drugs produce alertness and a sense of well-being, reduce appetite and cause insomnia. Frequent use can cause paranoia, aggressiveness and physical symptoms including damage to the nose through regular "snorting." Users of large quantities can develop a form of schizophrenia. Tolerance to these drugs develops quickly, so the user requires larger and larger doses and may be in for a rough time when next requiring dental treatment. Withdrawal symptoms include extreme fatigue and depression.

Heroin and other narcotic drugs induce a feeling of peace (narcosis) in users, so that they cease to suffer emotional or physical anguish. Narcotics reduce aggression and the desire for sex and food. Regular users tend to lose interest in everything except making sure they get supplies of their drug. Addiction to heroin develops remarkably quickly, particularly if high doses are taken, and withdrawal is every bit as bad as is claimed; the need for the drug can destroy addicts physically and socially. Users find they need rapidly escalating doses in order to achieve the same effects. When the drug is not available, craving for it and withdrawal symptoms develop within hours. These symptoms typically include restlessness, nausea, chills, cramps, pain in the back, abdomen and legs, and gooseflesh (hence "going cold turkey" as the term for heroin withdrawal).

The top of the addictive pyramid is currently held by *crack*. This is a cocaine derivative which is described as "instantly addictive." Its effects are described as a prolonged orgasm in the mind, a rapid high followed by a deeper low. Crack has become a major problem in many cities throughout the United States; its distribution is associated with a frightening level of violence. Unfortunately, because of the prevalence of cocaine, the ease of crack production, and the intense effects of the drug, it is a problem that will not be readily solved.

To summarize: our society is one in which drugs are difficult to avoid. Whether they are the illicit addictive substances associated with crime and social breakdown, the prescribed pharmaceuticals used for illness, over-the-counter medications, condoned recreational drugs, substances we consider as foods, the chemicals we put in foods, or the residues of the chemicals we use to grow and process that food, all have some action on our minds and bodies which may or may not be desirable. Against this background it is understandable that the main thrust of conventional medicine is based upon drugs. Our attitudes toward them make their use entirely compatible with our wider social ethic. It may also be understandable that many young people see little wrong with experiments or addiction to illicit drugs. When children see parents dying for a cup of tea, unable to function without coffee or desperate to distraction for a drink or a cigarette, how or why should they distinguish between this behavior and the use of pot, glue or heroin? Simply to say that it is wrong, legally or morally, is not enough, and to claim that such drugs are bad for health, implying that others are good, will not wash either. Children are not born with the same assumptions as their parents.

The social grounds on which we deprecate certain drugs are also invalid. Politicians may believe that heroin, cocaine and crack destroy hope and aspiration in young people, and seek to turn off the supply of such substances. Logic, however, suggests the opposite: it is because many young people have no hope, no outlet for their energy and aspirations, that they turn to drugs.

So what should our attitude to drugs be? The ideal, rational approach is to use drugs, of whatever sort, *only* when their effects are fully understood and desired. Increasingly we have the choice of realizing this ideal and avoiding undesirable and damaging drugs.

PART 2

CONDITIONS AND OPTIONS

4

Emotional Distress and Mental Illness

This chapter deals with depression, anxiety, neurosis, panic, stress, phobias, obsessions, insomnia and schizophrenia.

Depression is very common. It is particularly likely to affect adolescents and young adults, especially those who do not have jobs outside the home; young mothers are the most vulnerable group. The problem peaks again among the middle-aged; it is often part of the "mid-life crisis" experienced by both men and women, and it can recur among the elderly, especially the widowed. Doctors report that the people who are most likely to consult them with symptoms of depression are women between the ages of twenty-five and forty-four.

Depression usually clears up of its own accord within a year, but it may recur. A minority of sufferers experience extreme mood swings, from elation and hyperactivity (mania) to depression.

Depression is associated with greatly increased vulnerability to illness and with risk of death from suicide.

Anxiety affects all of us from time to time, but its more extreme manifestations (dubbed "neurosis" by doctors) are most likely to occur among mature adults, especially women aged forty-five to sixty-four. Excessive anxiety can develop a self-perpetuating momentum.

Phobias and obsessions are linked with anxiety. They may last indefinitely and can get steadily worse unless action is taken to curb them.

Insomnia is usually a symptom of anxiety or depression. It is likely to disappear spontaneously when the underlying problems are solved.

Schizophrenia most often develops among young adults, and is more likely to affect men than women. It can start insidiously or with a sudden, dramatic breakdown. It is usually recurrent but sometimes it occurs only once or twice in a lifetime. While it is usually episodic, with swings from relative normality to acute and obvious abnormality, it can be chronic, fluctuating little from day to day or even from year to year. Complete spontaneous recovery is rare.

The main difficulty with emotional illness is that of distinguishing between normality and abnormality, sanity and madness, transient difficulty and illness. The conditions listed above are not clear-cut or closely defined; they represent variations from what we in this society see as normal. Emotionally disturbed people typically cannot make rational judgments about their own condition, and the point at which the distressed person is acknowledged to be ill and in need of treatment varies according to the perspective of the observer. Inevitably there is great variation in opinion as to who should be treated and what form such treatment should take.

The pain of personal unhappiness drives a great many people to consult their doctors, who predominantly offer drug therapy. Some patients continue to take mind-altering (psychoactive) *drugs for year upon year, but these medicines can cause a host of problems which may not have been recognized when treatment began. Tranquilizers and sedatives are now accepted to be addictive; millions have become addicts, gaining no real benefit yet unable to tolerate the misery of breaking their habit.*

Emotional problems represent the second most common reason for consultation in general practice and they are undoubtedly the most important underlying reason for illness in the community. Frequently they coexist with, and indeed often precipitate, other forms of health breakdown. They therefore need to be taken seriously. Individual action may be possible but it will not be sufficient if the problem is too great.

SECTION INDEX

4.1 *The mind and the brain: how they work*
4.2 *Depression*
4.3 *Drugs for depression*
4.4 *Alternatives to drugs for depression*
4.5 *Anxiety, neurosis, panic and stress*
4.6 *Drugs for stress symptoms*
4.7 *Alternatives to drugs for stress symptoms*
4.8 *Insomnia*
4.9 *Drugs for insomnia*
4.10 *Alternatives to drugs for insomnia*
4.11 *Schizophrenia*
4.12 *Drugs for schizophrenia*
4.13 *Alternatives to drugs for schizophrenia*
4.14 *Organizations which help with mental and emotional problems*

4.1 THE MIND AND THE BRAIN: HOW THEY WORK

At a physical level the brain is an electrochemical system which is constantly processing information from a wide range of sources. It monitors everything that goes on in the body, bringing problems and experiences to the conscious mind when they are judged significant by subconscious selection processes. It sorts and filters the wealth of information that is constantly being received by our sense organs. All this input is evaluated and interpreted in the light of experience. What we actually perceive is a manageable synthesis created by the mind.

This immensely complicated system is affected by influences ranging from the chemical to the spiritual; every part of our life is involved, individual and social, practical and theoretical. When any part of the system changes, other parts will be affected. Thus an alteration in brain biochemistry can affect mood, and vice versa; and an alteration in thought patterns can change hormonal influences, and vice versa. The scope for deliberate or unwitting change is enormous. Philosophers, scientists, mystics, healers, writers and musicians are still exploring our potential, for its boundaries are unknown.

The mind requires a high level of integration and consistency; our belief systems, actions and experiences must all fit together to produce a coherent whole. In some cases the personal fit is produced by what observers might call delusion, and a pattern that deviates very dramatically from what is usual in society will be labeled insanity. Sometimes the need for consistency produces intense discomfort. For example, a person who has had many setbacks may come to feel worthless even though the misfortune resulted from no personal fault; this self-image produces consistency.

Mood, thought, behavior and biochemistry adapt to and interact with changing circumstances. On the biochemical level, function is related to activity at the connections between the nerves that make up the brain. These work through the release of specialized chemicals at the nerve endings which set up electrical impulses in adjoining nerves. The availability of these chemicals (known as neurotransmitters) plays an important role in determining the ease with which impulses travel through the system concerned. For example, the system that makes us fall asleep depends on a substance called serotonin. If serotonin levels are raised by diet or drugs we tend to feel sleepy; if they fall too low, as in depression, we experience problems with sleep. Neurotransmitter activity fluctuates over the course of the day; each system has a cycle which is appropriate to our normal requirements. Serotonin levels tend to rise in the evening, falling during the night until they are no longer adequate to maintain sleep, at which point we wake up. Similarly the systems concerned with activity, muscular coordination and other aspects of day-to-day life will fluctuate as demands change.

We do not know how many different systems there are, nor much about the way they interact; but we do know enough now to understand that we can influence our emotional state and functions by altering the brain's biochemistry. Many of the alternatives to drug therapy described in this chapter use current knowledge of influences on brain chemistry to change experience and behavior.

4.2 DEPRESSION

Depression is "an emotional state of dejection and sadness ranging from mild discouragement and downheartedness to feelings of utter hopelessness and despair" (Andrew Stanway, *Overcoming Depression*). It can be a very serious condition which totally disrupts the sufferer's life and career and can lead to suicide. The characteristics of depression vary in different cultures, but in the West depressed people tend to suffer very low self-esteem, loss of interest in themselves, guilt, a sense of hopelessness and helplessness, slow thinking, poor memory and a wide range of bodily symptoms from constipation to inexplicable pain. They usually have problems with eating, sleeping (early-morning waking in particular) and sex. Sufferers neglect themselves; they are tearful, fearful and fretful, and many feel excessively tired and weak.

In children, bodily symptoms tend to predominate. Depression leads to poor appetite, headaches, weight loss, sleep problems, school problems, abdominal pains and crying. Depressed adolescents often become more rebellious, some turning to drugs or sexual promiscuity.

Depressed people have been found to have abnormally low levels of the neurotransmitters serotonin and norepinephrine in their brains, but whether this is a cause or an effect of depression is not known.

The duration of depression is very variable. Often it is a temporary

state. Even with serious depressive illness, spontaneous recovery will
usually occur within a year. For some people the problem recurs on a
regular cyclic basis; others are prone to depression whenever life
becomes difficult. Many women suffer intense spells of depression a
few days before each period (we deal with this along with other
premenstrual problems in chapter 14).

Depression is extremely common in our society and it is becoming
more so. There are a number of different causes, the most common
being stress that is too great to bear. Major life changes, bereavement
and loss of any type can cause depression. Usually it is short-lived but
it can become persistent, especially in a grieving person who lacks
social support or feels responsible for what has happened. Some
people have less ability to cope with these pressures than others;
vulnerable groups include the poor, the socially isolated, people who
lost their mothers during childhood and those who have depressed
family members. For about half of the women who complain of
depression, relationships with men seem to be at the root of the
problem. Those who have just had or lost a baby are also very
vulnerable. So are women who have had hysterectomies or other
major surgery and those who take oral contraceptives; hormone
changes make all of these women more than usually susceptible.

Certain drugs and illnesses also cause depression. It is common
after virus infections including flu and mononucleosis, and in people
with chronic debilitating or painful conditions. Over 200 different
drugs have been linked with depression; the most common are tranquilizers, sleeping tablets, alcohol, oral contraceptives and drugs
prescribed for heart and blood-pressure problems, Parkinson's disease, cancer and diabetes.

Finally, depression may result from allergies, particularly sensitivity to food, mold spores and chemicals. In these cases it may be
very difficult to isolate the cause unless there is a clear relationship
between feeling depressed and eating particular foods, being exposed
to particular substances or staying in particular buildings. It is a
possibility that should be considered if depression is recurrent or
chronic and seems not to be linked with any of the factors mentioned
above. Detailed descriptions of such cases are given in *Eating Dangerously* by Dr. Richard Mackarness. (See chapter 6 for more information on allergies.)

4.3 DRUGS FOR DEPRESSION

The drugs that doctors most often prescribe for depression fall into two major groups: antidepressants and tranquilizers. Tranquilizers (see section 4.6) and sleeping tablets (section 4.9) are often prescribed for depressed people but they can sometimes make the condition worse. Suppressing grief with such drugs often extends the period of grieving and interferes with normal recovery; however, tranquilizers may be useful in the very short term to help a bereaved person to cope with funeral and other arrangements.

The drugs in the first two of the following lists are antidepressants. There are two major types, with differing effects and side effects: tricyclic antidepressants and related drugs, and monoamine oxidase inhibitors. The third drug, lithium, is a toxic mineral with quite different effects.

(a) Tricyclic antidepressants and related drugs

Amitriptyline (Elavil, Endep); desipramine (Norpramin, Pertofrane); doxepin (Adapin, Sinequan); imipramine (Tofranil); maprotiline (Ludiomil); nortriptyline (Pamelor); protriptyline (Vivactil); trazodone (Desyrel); trimipramine (Surmontil).

Compound antidepressants, containing both drugs from the list above and tranquilizers, include Libritol, Etrafon and Triavil.

Antidepressants act by raising the levels of the particular neurotransmitters in the brain which are generally reduced in depression, thus reducing the severity of the symptoms. They do not affect the underlying problems. While they may help you to feel better, they are not actually necessary, and the proportion of people who improve with antidepressant drug treatment is only about 20% more than the proportion who improve with placebos. Many types of nondrug therapy used by psychologists and psychotherapists give equally good or better results without the risk of serious adverse effects or addiction.

Tricyclic antidepressants take about two weeks to produce their effects. Side effects include dry mouth, sedation, fuzzy thinking, blurred vision, constipation, nausea, difficulty with urination, low blood pressure, fast heartbeat, sweating, tremor, rashes, weight gain, confusion (particularly in the elderly), behavior disturbances (particularly in children) and interference with sexual function. Less common side effects include blood disorders, convulsions and jaundice. These drugs should not be taken by people with heart disease because they have been linked with fatal disturbance of heart rhythm.

(b) Monoamine oxidase inhibitors (MAOIs)

Isocarboxazid (Marplan); phenelzine (Nardil); tranylcypromine (Parnate).

Like the tricyclic antidepressants, these drugs alter the levels of neurotransmitters, though by a different biochemical route which produces a different range of risks and side effects. Monoamine oxidase inhibitors can cause a very dangerous increase in blood pressure through interaction with chemicals in certain foods, drinks and medicines. When taking any of these drugs, and for fourteen days after taking them, you must not eat or drink any of the following: cheese, pickled herring, broad-bean pods, meat or yeast extract, Chianti wine and certain drugs including tricyclic antidepressants and medicines bought without prescription. Ask your pharmacist if you are in any doubt.

Side effects of this group include dizziness, agitation, headache, tremor, insomnia, constipation, dry mouth, blurred vision, urination problems, liver damage and rashes.

(c) Lithium

Lithium carbonate (Eskalith, Lithane, Lithobid); lithium citrate (Cibalith-S).

When depression is part of a pattern of dramatic mood cycles going from excessive stimulation and euphoria (mania) to bleak depression, the mineral lithium may be prescribed. Lithium has no value in the treatment of existing depression; it can sometimes prevent it but will not cure it. It is occasionally used when the euphoric or manic phase does not develop, in the hope of preventing the onset of depression. The concentration of the drug in the blood must be monitored because lithium is a toxic mineral; blood tests should be done at least once a month. Fits, coma and death can result from overdosage. Side effects include stomach problems, excessive appetite and weight gain. Intoxication, tremor, drowsiness and giddiness are signs that the dose is too high. Hormone and kidney changes, leading to serious metabolic symptoms, can also occur.

4.4 ALTERNATIVES TO DRUGS FOR DEPRESSION

Severely depressed people feel unable to help themselves. They cannot "pull themselves together." The hopelessness, lack of energy and loss of motivation which are part of the condition inevitably interfere with any efforts to overcome it through individual action. Family and friends may be able to encourage and persuade a depressed person to embark on self-help, but they may have to carry a heavy burden if they want to help lift the depression. It often seems like a thankless task which drags those who care into the same pit of despair. Nevertheless, the knowledge that someone does care deeply will be of great benefit and will undoubtedly reduce the risk that the depression will end in suicide.

Fortunately, few depressed people are down all the time. Usually the severity of the problem fluctuates, with some good days and some dreadful days. Taking action to alleviate the depression on the good days will help prevent the mood from swinging down so far next time, and recovery will gradually accelerate.

Depression-prone people can recognize the threat of a downswing. As storm clouds gather on the horizon, determined action at this point can prevent the development of the problem. It is important not to ignore warning mood changes, because the onset of anxiety or loss of self-confidence will make you reluctant to look after yourself; at this time it is imperative that you treat yourself as well as you possibly can.

One useful approach to depression is based on the idea that by changing the way you *behave* you can change the way you *feel*. This goes for all aspects of behavior. For example, if you move slowly when depressed, moving fast will tend to improve your mood; similarly, adopting the posture associated with cheerfulness and confidence— head high, shoulders straight, no slumping—will make you feel more cheerful.

Those who are caring for a depressed person should discourage depressive behavior with persuasion. For example, don't allow self-neglect; coax your depressed relative or friend to wash and dress attractively, to eat well and to go out. Involving depressed people in social and physical activities is very valuable, but it is often best to spring such activities on them with little warning, for they may fear and reject anything that seems at all unusual or potentially demanding.

Since guilt and self-blame are so much part of depression, it is essential that the depressed person is not punished or blamed for failing to behave in the desired way. Warm approval for progress will help, and talking is also very beneficial. A trained outsider such as a counselor or psychologist will usually be able to do more than family or friends, but anyone and everyone can help by including the depressed person in conversation, listening and giving permission to vent anger or express grief. It is important not to dismiss or make light of the depressed person's worries, nor to change the subject when something painful comes up. These worries must be aired, though it may be possible to persuade the depressed person not to feel so responsible for things that have gone wrong in the past, and to accept the possibility that the future could be better.

It is particularly important to encourage a bereaved person to talk about the one who has died. If you want to help someone to get over grief, offer a sympathetic shoulder to cry on—don't try to cut short the crying.

Regular association with other people is valuable for both alleviating depression and reducing susceptibility to it. Having a job is usually helpful, but if your depression makes it difficult to cope with the sort of work you might normally do, try to find something less challenging, such as community or environmental work. Carers can sometimes find opportunities for depressed people which they would not discover for themselves. Once they are established in a regular useful role, however, their ability will return to former levels.

Voluntary organizations can provide niches for depressed people who are not able to hold down paid employment; volunteer work can be ideal. Being a member of any active group—whether it be your local church, women's or environmental group—will help ward off depression. You may find that it helps to talk with others who have been through similar experiences; some useful addresses are given at the end of this chapter.

Depression in one or both members of a couple is very often the result of marital or relationship problems. Ask yourself if your depression might be linked with an unsatisfying relationship; if the answer could be yes, make an appointment with a counselor for help in sorting out your difficulties.

Insomnia, anxiety, agitation and fretfulness are commonly associated with depression. For strategies that will help alleviate these aspects of the problem, see sections 4.7 and 4.10.

Activity helps alleviate depression, while fairly demanding physical activity such as swimming or jogging can produce long-term significant improvements in mood. It may be useful for the depression-prone to know that strenuous activity produces marked changes in brain neurotransmitter levels. Serotonin, the transmitter involved in sleep, rises by 20% after swimming to exhaustion; and since low levels of serotonin are the likely cause of the early-morning wakefulness that so plagues depressed people, swimming or jogging for as long as you can may be sufficient to cure this problem. (See chapter 17, particularly sections 17.3, 17.4 and 17.7.)

Most depressed people make their condition worse by their lack of interest in a healthy diet. A good diet can help to alleviate the problem; conversely, an unbalanced diet will tend to make it worse. Complex carbohydrate foods (whole grains and vegetables) are particularly beneficial, while meat can help some sufferers. Try to avoid sugar. Vitamin B_6 supplements can relieve some forms of depression; a dose of 50 mg. every day will do no harm and may solve the problem.

4.5 ANXIETY, NEUROSIS, PANIC AND STRESS

Anxiety can be chronic and generalized, an ever-present sense of apprehension or nameless dread, or it can take the form of acute episodes which occur spontaneously or in response to particular things or events. Acute anxiety results in panic attacks. Symptoms include palpitations, rapid thumping heartbeat, chest pain, dizziness, faintness, problems with breathing, sweating, shaking, choking and weakness in the limbs. Many sufferers who experience these symptoms believe that they could be having a heart attack, even that they are dying. Because intense fear puts strain on the heart, panic attacks can sometimes cause heart problems, but worrying about your heart will only increase your anxiety level and make matters worse. To deal with all these problems you must learn how to reduce your anxiety level.

Panic attacks related to exposure to specific situations or objects are symptoms of phobias or irrational fears. If you are so terrified of spiders, cats, snakes or germs that you panic when confronted with them, you may be phobic. The most common type is agoraphobia, which is associated with panic attacks in public places or indeed anywhere outside the home. Claustrophobia, the fear of being trapped, is also common; it may be manifested as fear of traveling in airplanes, elevators or subways, or of being trapped in meetings or other situations from which rapid escape is difficult.

Obsessions and compulsions are forms of adaptation to severe anxiety. They entail the repeated and irrational need to take some particular form of action, commonly hand-washing. Sufferers may wash their hands or check the locks on their houses or perform some other ritual many times in the day; if they fail to do it they become extremely anxious.

Neurosis is the general term used by the medical profession for these problems. They are all aspects of the more general problem of emotional stress. The unpleasant sensations experienced by sufferers are manifestations of the hormonal changes caused by stress. The rapid, pounding heartbeat, for example, is part of the "fight or flight" pattern of reaction, but its hazards and unpleasantness are compounded by responses to fear, particularly rapid, shallow breathing which upsets the biochemical balance of the blood and produces faintness, breathlessness and other symptoms such as chest pain. Symptoms often begin at times of increased demands—for example, after changing jobs, moving or after a period of difficulties in the family or at work. Exhaustion and depression increase susceptibility to stress symptoms. (See chapter 9 for more information about symptoms.)

4.6 DRUGS FOR STRESS SYMPTOMS

The "minor" tranquilizers are most often prescribed, including alprazolam (Xanax); chlordiazepoxide (Librax, Librium); chlormezanone (Trancopal); clonazepam (Klonopin); clorazepate (Tranxene); diazepam (T-Quil, Valium, Valrelease); hydroxyzine (Atarax, Marax, Neucalm, Vistaril); lorazepam (Ativan); meprobamate (Deprol, Equagesic, Equanil, Meprospan, Miltown, PMB 200, PMB 400); oxazepam (Serax); prazepam (Centrax).

These drugs, with the exception of meprobamate and hydroxyzine, are benzodiazepines, a group of which the best-known member is Valium. They reduce muscle tension and induce relaxation and sleep. Once regarded as very safe, they have been prescribed more often than any other drugs. Their main danger is that they cease to be effective after some weeks of continuous use; tolerance and addiction develop. Withdrawal can induce symptoms ranging from those for which they were originally taken (though often worse) to madness—a full-blown toxic psychosis. Barbara Gordon's *I'm Dancing as Fast as I Can* gives a graphic account of this experience.

Side effects of benzodiazepines include drowsiness, dizziness, problems with walking (especially in the elderly), confusion, dry mouth, headache and hypersensitivity. They can also cause "paradoxical effects"—excitement, aggression and anger. Like alcohol, which exacerbates these effects, they can release violent or antisocial behavior.

Meprobamate is similar to the benzodiazepines but less effective and more addictive, with more frequent side effects.

Doctors who are disillusioned with tranquilizers are increasingly prescribing beta blockers such as propranolol (Inderal, etc.). Beta blockers are considerably more dangerous than benzodiazepines (see section 9.3(*a*)). Alternatively, some doctors prescribe low doses of drugs used for schizophrenia (see section 4.12), though these too can have very serious side effects, especially in the elderly. Tricyclic antidepressants (section 4.3) may also be given, particularly to phobic patients.

The trouble with taking tablets for problems of this sort is that they can offer only temporary benefit. They may be entirely appropriate for people who confront the situation they fear quite rarely—for example, air travel or dentists—but for agoraphobics and sufferers from generalized anxiety they can do more harm than good because the condition is likely to continue indefinitely unless action is taken to deal with the problem at a different level.

Millions of people who started taking tranquilizers for problems of this sort are now addicted to them; they are in a sort of limbo where ceasing to take the tablets produces predictable and unmanageable panic (with associated physical symptoms such as abdominal pain), while the original condition is no longer alleviated. It's a vicious circle that's best avoided.

Withdrawal from tranquilizers has to be slow. Finding alternative ways of dealing with problems will help break the dependence, but you should not try to cope with addiction alone; enlist the aid of others who have freed themselves from it. Contact Drugs Anonymous (see end of chapter for address) for help if you have difficulty finding a local group.

4.7   ALTERNATIVES TO DRUGS FOR STRESS SYMPTOMS

The first step in overcoming stress problems is to understand their nature so that you worry less about them. This is especially important with panic attacks, which can be so frightening that they induce a general increase in tension.

Panic attacks, like all the problems we deal with in this section, are symptoms of general tension and anxiety. When tension reaches a critical point you begin to gasp for breath, and if your normal breathing has been rather shallow and rapid, as it is with many anxious people, further problems develop very rapidly. The solution is twofold: learn better breathing habits, and take positive action to reduce your general level of tension. Both these topics are discussed in detail in chapter 16.

If you can also see a way to reduce the stress under which you are living, perhaps by relinquishing some responsibilities or delegating tasks to someone else, then your chances of success will be enhanced. You may need to learn to say no more often, so that you have more time for relaxation.

(a) Relaxation

Relaxation often seems impossible to chronically anxious people. Do not be discouraged by the fact that you can't simply choose to relax; you can be taught to unwind and there are many systems and hints that will help. Read chapter 16 carefully and follow the suggestions there.

(b) Activity

Research has shown that rhythmic activity will of itself reduce muscle tension and it is very effective in controlling anxiety. Many people imagine that an emotional problem can be solved only through psychological techniques, but this is not true at all. It is a misconception that has grown up through our culture's separation of mind from body. In reality—as all those with emotional problems will recognize if they think about it—the state of the mind affects the body and the body in turn affects the mind. The two are inseparable. You can work on emotional problems by working your body. Read chapter 17, sections 17.1, 17.2, 17.4 and 17.7, for detailed advice.

(c) Diet

Irregular meals and poor nutrition make you more vulnerable to stress symptoms. Make sure you are getting the food you need when you need it by following the advice in chapter 18, sections 18.2, 18.3, 18.4(*b*), 18.5(*b*) and 18.9.

(*d*) Desensitization

This is a form of treatment developed by psychologists for phobias. The phobic person is taught to relax completely, then to confront the thing or situation that induces fear. Relaxation prevents the onset of panic, so with repeated exposure the fear gradually diminishes until it eventually disappears altogether.

If your phobia involves spiders, cats or other common creatures you can organize your own desensitization. But before you begin, you must learn deep relaxation. Use chapter 16 and find a yoga or relaxation teacher to help you. Once you know how to relax you can choose to relax yourself consciously and begin to study what it is that frightens you. If it is spiders, begin with books or videos on spiders. Get used to representations of them. Learn all you can about them. Then go into the garden and watch little spiders in the wild. Go closer and closer until you feel your fear returning—then retreat. Don't push yourself into a full-blown panic; a little mild anxiety is as far as you should go. Repeat your relaxation exercises at frequent intervals so you stay completely relaxed. Practice as often as you can; gradually you will find that you can get close to larger and larger spiders without feeling afraid. Eventually you will be able to touch a spider with only the merest shadow of fear, which will disappear soon enough.

This process can happen without any deliberate effort if you take holidays in a cottage where there are many spiders; we have known spider-phobics who have lost their fear completely after a move to the country where they encountered spiders frequently in a nonthreatening environment.

Desensitization for the most common phobia, agoraphobia, is easiest with the help of a patient, trusted friend or relative. If you don't have anyone with the patience to help you, try to get your doctor to refer you to a psychologist, though if you have mastered relaxation techniques thoroughly you may be able to do it alone. The key to success is learning to relax completely, and then confronting, very, very gradually, the situations you fear. Don't try to take desensitization too fast; at the first signs of panic, retreat into safety and practice your relaxation techniques again.

Your desensitization may have to start at your own front door. Practice going out with your friend, shutting the door behind you and walking as far as the street. Practice your relaxation method at your garden gate or at the end of your driveway. Then come in again and relax. Do this repeatedly till you no longer have any anxiety about going out that far. Then practice without your friend. Just go out the door, go to the street, turn around, walk back and let yourself into your house again. Make sure you are relaxed all the time.

Another day, when your friend comes again, go a little further, to the nearest shop, perhaps. You will have to judge how far you can go. Practice with your friend until you have lost your fear of this short journey. Then practice alone. Extend your journeys outside your home until you can go anywhere—but don't go too far before you are ready. You need to work this sort of fear out of your system very slowly and very gently. If you push yourself too hard, you will be back where you started.

If you find you have gone a bit too far or too fast, and the panic begins, think about your breathing. Breathe as slowly as you can. Ignore everything else; just breathe very slowly. The panic sensation will retreat. Chapter 16 gives more details on breathing; make sure you are thoroughly familiar with all that is written there.

Tewap (a for-profit organization) offers counseling for phobics, especially agoraphobia sufferers; the toll-free number is (800) 2-PHOBIA.

4.8   INSOMNIA

Insomnia means an inability to sleep. The problem may be either that you are unable to get off to sleep or that you wake too early in the morning. If you lie awake for hours before nodding off, read sections 4.5 and 4.7 on stress problems; if you doze off quite well but wake before dawn and are unable to get back to sleep, read sections 4.2 and 4.4 on depression. Depression, anxiety and pain (see chapter 12) are the most common underlying causes of sleeping problems, and the first course of action is to do whatever you can to reduce their severity.

Other common causes include the effects of drugs, particularly caffeine in coffee and strong tea, and hunger if you are on a restrictive diet. Disturbance by traffic, a restless partner, babies, light or noise can lead to a level of chronic sleep deprivation which produces tension and makes deep sleep progressively more elusive.

4.9 DRUGS FOR INSOMNIA

Drugs given for sleeping problems are called hypnotics or sedatives. They fall into four groups:

(a) Benzodiazepines

Flurazepam (Dalmane); temazepam (Restoril); triazolam (Halcion).

These products are basically the same as the tranquilizers discussed in section 4.6 above, and have the same side effects. Residual effects are common the following day, and repeated use can lead to accumulation of the drug in the body, increasing the risk of adverse effects and accidents. Addiction develops within a few weeks; the first sign is "rebound insomnia," when your sleeping problems get worse than ever if you fail to take the tablets.

(b) Chloral hydrate and related drugs

Chloral hydrate; dichloralphenazone (Isocom, Midrin).

These drugs are similar to the benzodiazepines in their effects. Side effects include rashes, confusion and stomach problems.

(c) Antihistamines

Promethazine (Phenergan); trimeprazine (Temaril).

See Section 6.4 for information on antihistamines. Drowsiness is generally regarded as an unwelcome side effect of antihistamine treatment for allergies, but these drugs are often used to induce sleep in children.

(d) *Barbiturates and methyprylone*

Butisol Sodium, Nembutal, Nodular, Pyridium Plus.

These drugs are little used today because they have long been known to induce addiction; withdrawal is very difficult and can be fatal. Barbiturate overdose has caused many deaths, and accidental overdose can result from drug-induced confusion.

All drugs used for insomnia have serious drawbacks: they are addictive; they reduce alertness the day after use and thus can cause accidents; and the quality of sleep they induce is often inferior to natural sound sleep.

4.10   ALTERNATIVES TO DRUGS FOR INSOMNIA

Before you plan your campaign for better sleep you should consider the possibility that you do not actually have a sleep problem. This is not as foolish as it may sound at first. Many people who believe that they suffer from insomnia do in fact get as much sleep as they need; the problem is that they believe they need more than they actually do. People vary widely in their need for sleep. If you are one of those who require only five or six hours a night, but you try to sleep for eight, you will find yourself lying awake. So judge your own needs on the basis of internal cues, not assumptions; if you are not at all tired at bedtime, perhaps you should stay up longer.

We tend to require less sleep as we grow older, and our sleep needs vary with the sort of work we do. We find that we need more sleep when our days are filled with intellectual as opposed to physical activity. Some people, particularly the elderly, find that they do better with a shorter night and an afternoon nap. (This sleeping pattern is commonplace in Mediterranean cultures; many people in the United States could benefit from adopting the siesta habit.) In one old people's home the inmates were regularly given tablets to help them sleep at night. Then bedtime was put back two hours, and this simple change in routine virtually eliminated the need for drugs! The old people were thought to require tablets simply because they were expected to fall asleep too early. Staff convenience and expectations were at the root of the problem.

If you do wake in the night, or you find you cannot get to sleep when you go to bed, it may be unwise to lie there hoping to sleep. If you feel relaxed in the warmth of your bed and you are quite content there, then by all means stay; but if you start to feel frustrated and restless, get up. Have a snack (cereal and milk or yogurt is particularly appropriate), then read, write down the ideas that keep running around in your mind, listen to music or do relaxation exercises. Wait until you feel sleepy again before returning to bed.

Noise, light, a restless partner and other forms of distraction should be dealt with appropriately. Use soft wax earplugs to shut out sound, and reduce light with heavy curtains or an eye-shield. If your partner wakes you, you may have to sleep in a separate bed when you start to get overtired; alternatively, a mattress that does not spread vibration throughout the bed when one person turns over could help you both to sleep. In some European countries double beds have two separate mattresses on them, side by side. This seems much more sensible than the conventional double mattress.

Specific dietary measures can enhance sleep, while certain common eating and drinking habits detract from it. These are the rules for anyone with sleeping problems:

1. If you like to drink late in the evening, choose a warm milk drink or a relaxing herb tea such as camomile. Avoid tea and coffee for *four hours* before you go to bed. These beverages contain stimulant drugs (see chapter 3) which will tend to keep you awake. In addition they make your kidneys work faster and therefore make you more likely to wake up because you need to urinate during the night.
2. A single drink of alcohol can help you to sleep, but more than this often interferes with sleep. Never have more than a small quantity of alcohol late in the evening.
3. Eat a high-carbohydrate meal or snack two hours before retiring.

A baked potato with a sprinkling of finely grated hard cheese is ideal. This will tend to raise the level of the neurotransmitter serotonin which is necessary for sound sleep. Avoid meat or eggs within three hours of going to bed because this will have the opposite effect.

4. Make sure that you do not go to bed hungry, and if you wake through hunger, get up and eat a yogurt and cereal snack or a cheese sandwich. Low-calorie diets cause sleeping problems.

Gentle activity at night will help to relax your muscles and aid sound sleep. An evening stroll could be enough; yoga would be better. Sex (masturbation if you don't have a partner) is often very good. Or make up your own routine of stretching exercises, reaching and bending your limbs and back. Follow with deep breathing and relaxation. (See section 16.6 for deep relaxation methods.)

If you find that restlessness, twitching or uncomfortable legs keep you awake, activity followed by specific exercises to stretch the backs of the legs will help. Sit on the floor with your legs out in front of you as straight as possible, and pull your toes toward your head, bending as far as possible at the ankle. You will feel the strain in the backs of your legs. Pull and hold for ten seconds; relax; repeat five times. Then, lying on your back, lift your legs to a vertical position and hold them there for one minute. This will relieve the congestion in the veins that often causes restless legs.

Most conducive of all to sound sleep is a relaxed mind. We describe some methods of achieving this in chapter 16. Here are some more tips:

1. If you have to work in the evening, make sure you give yourself enough time to wind down before bed. You may need three hours free from mental concentration before sound sleep is possible.
2. Reading is better than TV for presleep relaxation—but don't choose a book that is so exciting that you won't be able to put it down!
3. Music can be very calming. Choose your record or tape carefully; you don't want one that will make you want to jump up and bop about, or one that tells of great passions and disasters!

4.11   SCHIZOPHRENIA

Schizophrenia is the name given to a pattern of symptoms of mental and behavioral breakdown which can take a variety of forms. Sufferers show disorders of thought and speech, and are prone to delusions—of personal power or persecution or of changed identity—and hallucinations, usually voices. They feel isolated and seem to lack normal emotional responses, but may be profoundly fearful of the process that is going on inside them. They can be withdrawn or garrulous, apathetic or hyperactive. The onset of the condition can be acute and dramatic or gradual, and it can be episodic or chronic in nature. Sometimes it occurs only once or twice in a lifetime, but it is usually recurrent.

The cause of schizophrenia is unknown. Susceptibility runs in families, and biochemical abnormalities have been found in the brains of schizophrenics, though it is not known whether these are cause or effect. Schizophrenia often seems to be linked with psychological and social stress, and it is most likely to develop for the first time in early adulthood.

Stimulant drugs such as amphetamine and cocaine, and hallucinogenic drugs, notably LSD, can precipitate schizophrenic breakdown, especially if they are used in high doses over a period of weeks or more. Food allergies may also be capable of precipitating it.

4.12   DRUGS FOR SCHIZOPHRENIA

Drugs used to treat schizophrenia are known as antipsychotics, neuroleptics or "major" tranquilizers. They include: chlorpromazine (Thorazine); chlorprothixene (Taracton); droperidol (Inapsine, Innovar); fluphenazine (Permitil, Prolixin); haloperidol (Haldol); perphenazine (Etrafon, Triavil, Trilafon); pimozide (Orap); prochlorperazine (Compazine); promazine (Sparine); thioridazine (Mellaril); trifluoperazine (Stelazine).

Antipsychotic drugs reduce reactions to all types of stimulation, producing a state of emotional quietness and indifference. They can be given in tablet form or by injection. The effects of long-lasting injections continue for some weeks, the precise time depending on the drug and the individual patient.

One of the most troublesome side effects is a condition akin to Parkinson's disease, with abnormal movements and restlessness. This can usually be controlled with anti-Parkinson drugs such as orphenadrine (Disipal), benztropine (Cogentin), biperiden (Akineton) and procyclidine (Kemadrin). However, these can exacerbate the other major side effect of antipsychotics—tardive dyskinesia, characterized by uncontrollable movements, especially of the face, mouth and tongue. Tardive dyskinesia, which is untreatable and may be irreversible, can occasionally occur even after short-term treatment with low doses of antipsychotic drugs.

These drugs are particularly dangerous for the elderly because they interfere with temperature control, increasing the risk of hypothermia, and they blunt the reactions, making falls more likely. Other side effects include drowsiness, apathy, nightmares, depression, dry mouth, constipation, nasal congestion, blurred vision, low blood pressure and problems with heart rhythm, menstrual disturbances, breast swelling, weight gain, blood disease, excessive sensitivity to sunlight, rashes, liver disease, eye disease and purple blotches on the skin.

Many schizophrenics are put on maintenance therapy, which is continued indefinitely, usually with "depot" injections given at intervals. It is said that this prevents relapse, though the evidence for this is shaky; some schizophrenics have no recurrences even in the absence of drug therapy, while others will relapse in spite of it.

4.13 ALTERNATIVES TO DRUGS FOR SCHIZOPHRENIA

During the acute phase of schizophrenic breakdown, the only alternative to drugs is likely to be electroconvulsive therapy (ECT), also known as electroshock therapy. Psychotherapy is useful when the schizophrenic is able to make meaningful contact with other people, and it can help him to find his identity and reenter life in the community. In the long term it is helpful if the schizophrenic can take regular employment with other people, as this tends to keep him in touch with reality. Therapeutic communities have proved very valuable for schizophrenics.

Stress, both emotional and physiological, seems to be involved in schizophrenic breakdown, and avoidance of potentially stressful situations will tend to protect the schizophrenic from relapse. A regular life, with prompt attention to any potential sources of emotional demand and straightforward interactions between the schizophrenic and those who live with him, seems to offer the best hope for recovery. (See chapter 16 for advice on stress reduction.)

Keeping on an even emotional keel is easier if physiological and metabolic fluctuations are minimized. The adoption of a health-enhancing life-style, with regular physical activity (see chapter 17), an adequate balanced diet (see chapter 18) and rest when appropriate, will help.

Some doctors believe that schizophrenia can be due to food intolerance (see section 18.8). A gluten-free diet—one that contains no cereal or grain products—has been found to reduce the severity of schizophrenic symptoms in some patients. At the University Hospital in Philadelphia, Dr. Curtis Dohan found that schizophrenic patients who had never left the ward since the onset of their illness were able to go home or out to work once they were established on a cereal-free diet.

4.14   ORGANIZATIONS WHICH HELP WITH MENTAL AND EMOTIONAL PROBLEMS

American Association for Counseling and Development, 5999 Stevenson Ave., Alexandria, VA 22304. (703) 823-9800. Professional body of qualified counselors.

Compassionate Friends, P.O. Box 3696, Oak Brook, IL 60522. For parents who have lost a child.

Depression after Delivery, P.O. Box 1282, Morrisville, PA 19067. (215) 295-3994. Support for women with postpartum adjustment problems, depression or psychosis.

Depressives Anonymous: Recovery from Depression, 329 E. 62nd St., New York, NY 10021. (212) 689-2600. Self-help for people suffering from depression or anxiety.

Drugs Anonymous, P.O. Box 473, Ansonia Station, New York, NY 10023. (212) 874-0700. Helps addicts of all drugs including prescribed medicines.

Emotional Health Anonymous, 2420 San Gabriel Blvd., Rosemead, CA 91770. (818) 573-5480. Fellowship of people to help each other grow emotionally and spiritually; helps during and after a crisis.

Emotions Anonymous, P.O. Box 4245, St. Paul, MN 55104. (612) 647-9712. Network of regional groups assisting with recovery from mental illness.

International Association for Widowed People, P.O. Box 3564, Springfield, IL 62708. (217) 787-0886. Helps the widowed.

International Post-Partum and Mental Health Social Support Network, 927 N. Kellog Ave., Santa Barbara, CA 93101. (805) 967-7636. Aims to establish self-help groups for women with emotional problems after childbirth.

National Alliance for the Mentally Ill, 1901 N. Fort Myer Dr., Suite 500, Arlington, VA 22209. (703) 524-7600. Alliance of self-help/advocacy groups for the severely or chronically mentally ill. Support and guidance for families.

National Depressive and Manic-Depressive Association, 222 S. Riverside Plz., Chicago, IL 60606. (312) 993-0066. Offers support for sufferers and their families.

Neurotics Anonymous, P.O. Box 4866, Cleveland Park Station, Washington, DC 20008. (202) 232-0414. Helps emotionally ill people to recover.

Panic Attack Sufferers' Support Group, P.O. Box 1614, Williamsville, NY 14221. (716) 689-4399. Telephone counseling service manned by former sufferers.

Pills Anonymous, Box 459, Grand Central Station, New York, NY 10017. (212) 874-0700. For people addicted to pills.

Samaritans, 500 Commonwealth Avenue, Kenmore Sq., Boston, MA 02215. (617) 247-0220. Befriends the suicidal and depressed.

Schizophrenics Anonymous, 1209 California Rd., Eastchester, NY 10709. (914) 337-2252. Self-help organization for diagnosed schizophrenics.

Tewap, 1010 Doyle St., Menlo Park, CA 94025. (415) 329-1233. Offers information about phobias, especially agoraphobia; counseling for phobics. Toll-free number: (800) 2-PHOBIA.

Wives' Self-Help Foundation, Smylie Times Building, Suite 205, 8001 Roosevelt Blvd., Philadelphia, PA 19152. (215) 332-2311. Helps with marital, family and personal problems via PA-based hotline; provides information and referral.

5

Colds and Respiratory Infections

This chapter deals with respiratory infections and related problems including coughs, colds, sore throat, earache, flu, catarrh, sinus infections and bronchitis.

Respiratory infections are the most frequent reason for consulting doctors. Colds and sore throats are particularly common among children, while longer-lasting infections, especially bronchitis, predominantly affect the elderly. In the main these are minor annoyances to which we become accustomed; coughs and colds usually clear up quite quickly of their own accord. Long-lasting respiratory problems such as breathlessness and recurrent or perennial cold symptoms are often allergic in origin (see chapter 6).

All respiratory problems are much more common and more severe among smokers. Smoking both reduces resistance to colds, flu and bronchitis and increases their severity. Smokers are less able to throw off colds and are more susceptible to lingering effects. Whatever you smoke, you are likely to suffer some ill effects because you are irritating the delicate membranes of the respiratory passages; but the more you smoke and the more you inhale, the worse those effects will be. Children of smokers also suffer more respiratory infections.

SECTION INDEX

5.1   *The respiratory system*
5.2   *How we react to infections*
5.3   *Pain-relieving drugs*
5.4   *Sore throat remedies*
5.5   *Cold remedies*
5.6   *Cough mixtures*
5.7   *Antibiotics*
5.8   *Alternatives to drugs for colds and flu*
5.9   *Sore throat and tonsillitis*
5.10 *Earache*
5.11 *Coughs and bronchitis*
5.12 *Improving your immunity to infection*

5.1   THE RESPIRATORY SYSTEM

The respiratory system is designed to allow us to take in warm, filtered air, bring it down into the lungs where the oxygen is exchanged for carbon dioxide, and then breathe it out again. This process is essential for life because we need oxygen to burn our food and produce energy; but it is also a potential source of illness because the air contains many contaminants, from smoke and fumes to infectious organisms.

Air comes in through the nose and mouth, travels down the windpipe and then through two pipes called bronchi into the lungs. Specialized cells lining these passages protect us from the hazards in the air. These cells filter out airborne bacteria, viruses and other infectious organisms against which they have built-in defenses. They also remove most of the dust and other particles.

The membranes of our respiratory passages produce a layer of sticky mucus which traps unwanted material, and tiny hairs keep this mucus constantly moving away from the delicate internal surface of the lungs. Anything that gets through the mucus is assessed by mast cells which form the next line of defense in the respiratory membranes. They assess and identify the invader by comparing it with a "library" of information about potentially dangerous particles that each cell keeps on file. If the intruder is judged to be hazardous, a sequence of defensive reactions begins.

5.2   How we react to infections

The mast cells in the respiratory system respond to potential hazards by bursting, flooding the area with protective substances and setting up reactions in neighboring cells. If the invader is not eliminated immediately, more defense systems are mobilized.

Our immune systems have many levels which switch on one after another to protect us. Some are fast-reacting, like the interferons which are produced quickly in response to infection and which increase our cells' resistance to invasion by viruses, though they do not actually kill the infection; others are slower but more effective at killing enemy organisms. Interferons keep the infection at bay for a few days, giving our immune systems time to manufacture specific antibodies which are then used to mark and destroy bacteria and viruses. Once we have these antibodies available they can be produced every time we meet the infection for which they are specific; we become immune to it.

These reactions to infection, although effective in enabling us to survive a constant onslaught by an enormous range of bacteria, viruses and other microorganisms, do have some drawbacks. A massed reaction of respiratory mast cells results in sore and runny eyes and nose because one of the substances produced is an irritant, histamine. When an infecting organism penetrates deeper into our bodies we notice the effects of other protective systems. These are what we normally regard as the symptoms of illness; in fact they are more often signs that our bodies are fighting the illness. One of the effects of interferons is to make us feel feverish, headachy and unwell. This is actually beneficial to us because interferons work well when our body temperature is slightly raised, while most viruses prefer a lower temperature. So a raised temperature helps us to recover faster. If we feel tired, that too is entirely appropriate; when our bodies are using all available energy resources to combat infection, we should not be rushing around.

Infecting organisms are actually destroyed or gobbled up by white blood cells which can be mobilized in large numbers. These are mainly produced in our lymph glands, which swell up and may become quite prominent. This is why we sometimes notice swellings in our necks when we have a cold or other infection. White blood cells are also produced by our tonsils and certain other organs which may also swell, not necessarily because they themselves are infected but because they are actively involved in combating infection.

The all-too-familiar symptoms of upper respiratory infections can thus be understood in terms of the body's various ways of fighting infection. This has important implications for the way we deal with our symptoms; they may be unpleasant but they are not generally dangerous—rather the reverse. It is often true that by suppressing the symptoms with drugs we are interfering with our defenses against infection and possibly increasing the duration of the illness. For example, a raised body temperature is bad for viruses, which is why we tend to develop fever; reducing the temperature with medicines can therefore be better for the viruses, and while it may make us feel better for a while, it can cause the infection to last longer.

The majority of respiratory infections—coughs, colds, flu, acute bronchitis and pneumonia—are caused by viruses. These minute organisms invade the cells of our bodies and subtly pervert them so that they create millions more viruses instead of carrying on their normal functions. The viruses break out, leaving an empty cell behind. When someone with such an infection breathes out or, worse, sneezes, enormous numbers of viruses are released into the atmosphere to be breathed in by other people. Air-conditioned buildings which circulate the same air between large numbers of people provide a perfect environment for the spread of viruses; colds and other virus infections are more common today than at any time in the past.

5.3 PAIN-RELIEVING DRUGS

(a) Acetaminophen and combinations

Acetaco, Acetaminophen, Alba-Temp 300, Algisin, Anacin-3, Bancap HC, Beta-Phed, Bucet, Chexit, Codalan, Co-Gesic, Comtrex, Congespirin for Children, Coricidin, Datril, Dimetapp, Dolacet, Dorcol Children's Fever & Pain Reducer, Drixoral, Duocet, Esgic, Excedrin Fioricet, G-1 Capsules, Gelpirin, Liquiprin, Lorcet, Lortab, Lurline, Medigesic Plus, MegaMor, Midrin, Migralam, Panadol, Percocet, Percogesic, Phrenilin, Pyrroxate, Repan, Roxicet, Sedapap, Sinarest, Sine-Aid, Singlet, Sinubid, Sinulin, Sinutab, Sominex, Spasgesic, Supac, Talacen, Tempra, Tencet, Triad, Triminicin, Tylenol, Tylox, Unisom, Vanquish, Wygesic, Zydone.

Acetaminophen is America's most popular medicine. It is very safe when used occasionally, but you should not take it every day, as frequent use can lead to liver and kidney damage. While many preparations containing acetaminophen are available over the counter without a prescription, some products in the preceding list are available only with prescription. This is also generally true of combination products containing drugs which are not as safe as acetaminophen.

(b) Aspirin

Alka-Seltzer, Alpha-Phed, Anacin, Ascriptin, B-A-C Tablets, Bayer Aspirin, BC Powder, Bufferin, Carisoprodol, Easprin, Ecotrin, Empirin, Excedrin, Fiorinal, Gelpirin, Lortab ASA, Norgesic, Norwich Aspirin, Original Formula Midol, Percodan, Persistin, Robaxisal, Roxiprin, Soma Compound, Supac, Synalgos-DC, Ursinus, Vanquish, Zorprin.

Aspirin effectively reduces pain, inflammation and fever. Side effects are uncommon with low doses taken in accordance with instructions on the container. Nevertheless, aspirin and products containing aspirin should *never* be given to children because it has been linked with Reye's Syndrome, a disease that is often fatal.

Aspirin can cause stomach pain, nausea, vomiting and stomach bleeding. Guard against these problems by eating food before taking aspirin, by avoiding any combination of aspirin with alcohol and by taking soluble aspirin dissolved in water. Elderly, malnourished or debilitated people should avoid aspirin; they are particularly likely to react badly to it. Do not take aspirin if you have a peptic (stomach) ulcer, or if you use tablets for diabetes (see section 10.4(*a*)) or anticoagulants. Pregnant women should also avoid aspirin. Aspirin sensitivity is not unusual, especially among asthmatics.

(c) *Ibuprofen*

Ibuprofen is chemically similar to aspirin and has similar analgesic properties. It is not suitable for people who cannot take aspirin. Products containing ibuprofen include: Advil Ibuprofen, Haltran, Medipren, Midol 200, Motrin, Nuprin Ibuprofen, Rufen, Trendar.

Like aspirin, ibuprofen has such side effects as stomach problems, intestinal bleeding and allergic reactions.

5.4 SORE THROAT REMEDIES

Sore throat remedies contain a variety of ingredients. Some soothe discomfort through local anesthetic action—for example, Chloraseptic and Vicks Throat Lozenges; many contain traditional ingredients such as honey, lemon and licorice, which are generally harmless. Some contain antiseptics such as thymol; these are unlikely to offer any benefit but are also harmless unless you are unusually sensitive to them. Sucking a throat drop or lozenge will increase the production of saliva in your mouth, which will in turn soothe the inflamed surface of the throat.

5.5 COLD REMEDIES

This group includes a wide range of products with various mixtures of ingredients. Basically, most cold remedies contain one or more of three types of drug: a pain reliever (usually acetaminophen), decongestants and antihistamines. Decongestant sprays and nose drops are discussed in section 6.4(c).

Cold remedies containing acetaminophen and decongestant drugs include: Comtrex, Congespirin for Children, Contac, Coricidin D, Dimetapp, Drixoral, Pyrroxate, Robitussin, Sine-Off, Sinutab, Vicks Daycare, Vicks Formula 44, Vicks Nyquil.

Preparations containing antihistamines and decongestants include: Actifed, Alka-Seltzer Plus Cold Medicine, Allerest, Benadryl, Bromfed, Cerose-DM, Chlor-Trimeton, Comtrex Multi-Symptom Cold Reliever, Contac, Coricidin, Co Tylenol Cold Medication, Demazin, Dimetane, Dimetapp, Dristan, Drixoral, Fedahist, Novahistine, Pyrroxate, Robitussin Night Relief, Ryna Liquid, Sine-Off, Singlet, Sinutab, Sudafed, Triaminic, Trianimicol, Vicks Formula 44 Cough Mixture, Vicks Nyquil.

The addition of lemon and similar ingredients is mainly to increase palatability and fit in with popular folk remedies.

Cold remedies containing acetaminophen may relieve pain and inflammation, but see section 5.3, above, for other pain relievers. Decongestants can have serious side effects. They are particularly bad for people with stress problems, because they contain drugs (usually pseudoephedrine hydrochloride or phenylephrine hydrochloride) related to the natural hormone epinephrine, which stimulates the heart and increases blood pressure. It also dries up secretions in the respiratory membranes. Cold remedies can thus effectively mimic the dry mouth experienced with fear. Those who are sensitive to these drugs can suffer a hypertensive crisis, with very high levels of blood pressure. Cold remedies could theoretically precipitate a stroke or bleeding from delicate blood vessels such as those in the back of the eye, though to our knowledge this possibility has not been seriously investigated. If you suffer from any form of heart disease or diabetes, or if you take or have recently taken antidepressants of the MAOI group (see section 4.3(*b*)), you should not use these drugs.

Sprays and drops that you can put directly up your nose, such as Afrin Nasal Spray, Benzedrex Inhaler, Coricidin Decongestant Nasal Mist, Dristan, Duration 12 Hour Nasal Spray, 4-Way Nasal Spray, NT2, Neo-Synephrine, Nostril Nasal Decongestant, Otrivin, Privine and Vicks Sinex, also contain decongestant drugs. These can cause a chronically runny nose if they are used regularly. See section 6.4(c) for further warnings.

Most proprietary cold remedies contain antihistamines. Their main side effect is drowsiness but they can produce a range of other unwanted effects, from mood change to weight gain. Antihistamines have not been shown to help your body cope with respiratory infection, and they may actually make the illness worse because they interfere with the protective role of the mast cells.

5.6   COUGH MIXTURES

The cough reflex is the method the body uses to remove unwanted particles or substances from the respiratory passages. This is clearly necessary to us, though coughing that carries on for long periods without producing anything but discomfort is pointless.

Cough mixtures come in two major types: expectorants, which are said to increase the production of sputum, and cough suppressants, which act on the cough center of the brain to reduce the desire to cough. Some products contain a mixture of the two, which would seem totally irrational. Many include a cocktail of drugs; according to Professor Peter Parish, author of *Medicines: A Guide for Everybody*, "Some are useless, some are harmful, many are expensive, some are addictive, and it is difficult to find out what some of them contain." Many of the ingredients are the same as those in cold remedies (see section 5.5) and they share their dangers.

The opium derivative codeine and related narcotic (or sleep-inducing) drugs are effective cough suppressants; these drugs are generally restricted to prescription-only products because they can be addictive. Dextromethorphan is the main narcotic cough suppressant in cough mixtures available over the counter in the United States. Naldecon CX Adult Liquid, Ryna-C and Ryna-CX are examples of cough mixtures containing narcotic drugs. Their side effects may include delayed reactions and constipation. You should avoid driving and using machinery if you are taking a cough mixture.

5.7 ANTIBIOTICS

Antibiotics kill bacteria. They have no effect on viruses, which cause colds, sore throats and the vast majority of respiratory infections. Although a few doctors still prescribe them for sore throat and similar symptoms, experts now acknowledge that this is irrational and potentially dangerous.

Antibiotics upset the biological balance of the body and are capable of producing side effects, some of them serious. In addition, the more that antibiotics are used, the more resistant bacteria become to them. A large number of bacteria are now unaffected by the most popular types of antibiotic; if these powerful drugs continue to be overused, before long few of them will have any potency against bacteria.

Some of the more serious respiratory infections may be caused by bacteria, although these, too, can be viral in origin. Antibiotic treatment may be considered appropriate for pneumonia, bronchitis, earache and a limited range of other problems.

There are many types of antibiotics, the most common ones being penicillins, tetracyclines, co-trimoxazole and other sulphonamides.

(a) Penicillins

Amoxycillin (Amoxil, Augmentin, Trimox, Wymox); ampicillin (Omnipen, Principen, Unasyn); bacampicillin (Spectrobid); benzylpenicillin (Pre-Pen); cloxacillin; penicillin G (Bicillin, Pentids); penicillin V (Pen-Vee K, Veetids).

Penicillins are the safest antibiotics known. However, some people are sensitive to them and can suffer a very serious allergic reaction (anaphylaxis). If you get a rash when taking any of the drugs in this list, inform your doctor immediately and *never* take any form of penicillin again.

Bacterial resistance to penicillin is becoming increasingly common. These valuable antibiotics should never be taken casually. Take them as directed by your doctor and finish any course of tablets you start.

(b) *Tetracyclines*

Oxytetracycline (Terramycin, Urobiotic); tetracycline (Achromycin, Mysteclin, Sumycin, Topicycline).

These may be prescribed for bronchitis and other infections, though as with penicillin, resistant bacteria are now multiplying. Tetracyclines should not be used by children under twelve or by pregnant women, because they stain and damage developing teeth. Side effects include nausea, vomiting, diarrhea, infection with resistant organisms and fungi, and allergic reactions. Tetracyclines have also been linked with renal failure.

(c) *Co-trimoxazole and other sulphonamides*

Sulfamethizole (Thiosulfil, Urobiotic); sulfamethoxazole/Trimethoprim (Azo Gantanol, Bactrim, Ganatol, Septra, Sulfamethoprim); trimethoprim (Proloprim, Trimpex).

These are sometimes prescribed for chronic bronchitis and sinusitis. Side effects include nausea, vomiting, rashes and serious skin disorders, allergic reactions and many types of blood disease.

5.8 ALTERNATIVES TO DRUGS FOR COLDS AND FLU

Rational treatment of these common ailments requires some understanding of what is happening in your body when you suffer symptoms. It is obviously unwise to suppress symptoms which are part of the recovery process.

Many people believe they have flu when experts would diagnose an acute cold. Since the two conditions have many similar features, and both are caused by virus infections, the difference may be arbitrary and your approach should be the same whatever label the particular bug would be given in a laboratory. In the first phase of a virus infection the symptoms are subtle. You may feel a bit under par, with muscular aches; you may be tired and perhaps depressed; and your body's temperature-control systems may seem slightly awry, giving you hot flushes and a slight headache. These are signs that your cells are producing interferon, and by responding in a way that will help them you may be able to avoid developing a full-blown infection.

If you suspect you could be fighting an infection, it is not a good idea to override your malaise by taking medicines and drinking coffee so that you can carry on regardless. Work *with* your body. Attend to your health needs by making sure you are eating properly; have extra fresh fruit for vitamin C (especially oranges or other citrus and soft fruit—see section 18.4(f); drink plenty of pure water and/or fruit juice; keep warm and have early nights. Do *not* go running or undertake strenuous activity.

You may, however, succumb to the infection despite these precautions. The second stage of infection is more clear-cut, with symptoms that are all too familiar to most of us. Aches and pains, sneezes, sore throat, runny nose and fever are all characteristic of the common cold. Continue to work with your body to minimize the length of time you suffer. Don't just suppress the symptoms indiscriminately; they form part of the protective reaction. Instead of bringing down your fever with aspirin or acetaminophen you would be better advised to put up with it, at least for a day or so, to maximize your body's fighting power. Sweat it out. Keep warm even if you are sweating. If you feel tired, go to bed with a good book. Don't even consider going to work, school or meetings when you are in this highly contagious phase; you'll only spread the virus and retard your own recovery.

Drink plenty of fluid; fruit juice is particularly good, though you may find that hot drinks make you feel better. Try the traditional remedy: the juice of a fresh lemon and a teaspoon of honey diluted with hot water. Increase your intake of the anti-infection vitamin, vitamin C, by eating as much as you can of the foods listed in section 18.4(f).

There is some evidence that large doses of vitamin C can cut short the progress of a cold. This may not work for those who habitually eat enough fresh fruit and vegetables to get adequate dietary vitamin C, and research suggests that it is less likely to benefit women than men. But for most people there seems to be no harm in taking it for a few days since any excess is excreted in the urine. We are not convinced that the body can use synthetic ascorbic acid as readily as vitamin C from natural sources.

Use hot water vapor to ease problems with your nose and aid the body's fighting power at the nasal membranes. Fill a basin with boiling water, put a towel over your head, and breathe the steam— but take care you don't scald your nose! Menthol in the water may help clear your blocked passages.

Steam treatment is very useful for children's colds; steamy air will ease their symptoms and help them to breathe and recover. Let them play in a steamy bathroom or a kitchen in which a pot of water is boiling and close the doors and windows. But do ensure that they can't tip the pot over and scald themselves!

5.9 SORE THROAT AND TONSILLITIS

To ease a sore throat, gargle with a glass of warm water containing a teaspoon of salt. Don't swallow the solution. Repeat as often as you wish. A viral sore throat can persist for a week; don't bother to consult your doctor unless you also have a prominent skin rash, if you have had rheumatic fever or nephritis, or if you have a fever and thick yellow pus on the tonsils. If you still have a sore throat and feel unwell after a week, make an appointment to see your doctor; the cause may not be the common cold.

It is not always easy to see the tonsils in very young children, so look for the following symptoms: fever over 101°F or 38°C lasting twenty-four hours or more, swollen glands in the neck, headache and/or abdominal pain. If your child has this combination of symptoms, take him or her to see a doctor. *Never give a child aspirin in any form.* Aspirin has been linked with a serious disease called Reye's Syndrome which can develop when a child suffering from a virus is treated with aspirin.

5.10 EARACHE

Earache may be a transitory phenomenon associated with the acute phase of a cold, or it can develop after a cold when bacteria invade the vulnerable membranes of the ear. It is a problem that can return again and again. If the earache is severe you should consult a doctor without delay. Most doctors will prescribe antibiotics, usually some form of penicillin (see section 5.7(a)). Warn your doctor if you have ever had a skin rash or other signs of sensitivity to penicillin; you should remind him even if he knows you, because individual sensitivity is easily forgotten and an allergic reaction to penicillin can be very serious.

Unless your earache is mild and you are accustomed to occasional ear problems, you would be unwise to look for alternatives to antibiotic treatment. However, if you are one of those who develop earache very readily during or just after a head cold, you might know yourself well enough to feel you can tolerate the pain for a few hours, after which you may recover. Do not put up with it if you have discharge from the ear or if you feel generally ill and feverish. Consult a doctor. You won't need an appointment, since earache is recognized to be an urgent problem.

It is possible to ameliorate the pain of earache somewhat. Try a combination of heat close to the ear (a hot-water bottle is fine) and distraction. Watch a funny video or lose yourself in a novel. A hot bath may make you feel better. If you are susceptible to earache you can reduce the frequency of bouts by adopting the following strategies:

1. Give up smoking; ear infections often spread up the eustachian tubes from the throat, and smoking aggravates this problem.
2. Never go swimming when you have the least suggestion of a cold. Avoid getting water in your ears when washing your hair.
3. Don't clean inside your ears; they are self-cleansing and the wax has a protective function.
4. React quickly to any suggestion of a cold by looking after yourself, keeping warm, using steam inhalations and going to bed. Don't let it progress.

5.11 COUGHS AND BRONCHITIS

The cough reflex is another of the body's defense mechanisms. When your breathing tubes are irritated, obstructed or gummed up with mucus, the reflex is triggered in order to clear them. Coughing that brings up mucus is called "productive," and it should not be suppressed with medicines.

Chronic irritation of the bronchial tubes, such as that caused by smoking, can damage this mechanism, and the result is a dry cough. Smokers typically cough in the morning and the cough becomes more persistent as the damage increases through continued irritation. Eventually, chronic bronchitis develops.

Infection in the tubes can cause bleeding and the production of profuse thick yellow-green or brownish mucus. If you have these symptoms, and particularly if they are accompanied by a raised temperature and pain on breathing, you should consult a doctor. You could have acute bronchitis and need treatment.

Acute bronchitis is usually treated with antibiotics such as penicillin; if you have chronic bronchitis you may be given a longer course of a different type of antibiotic such as co-trimoxazole (see section 5.7(c) for brand names and further information). It is not wise to try to avoid taking antibiotics if your doctor confirms that you are suffering from acute bronchitis. You should finish the whole course of tablets; don't stop taking them just because you feel better, as the illness may recur if you do.

If you smoke, bronchitis is a warning you must heed. You cannot afford to continue smoking. You are seriously damaging your health. Antibiotics may get rid of the infection but it will return again and again and you could end up with serious lung disease. Bronchitis and chronic lung disease kill 75,000 people each year in the United States. Smoking is a major factor in most of these deaths. Contact these organizations for help with quitting cigarettes:

Action on Smoking and Health, 2000 H St., N.W., Washington, DC 20006. (202) 659-4310.
Five-Day Plan to Stop Smoking, Seventh-Day Adventist Church, Narcotics

Education Division, 6840 Eastern Ave., N.W., Washington, DC 20012.
(202) 723-0800.
SmokEnders, 3708 Mt. Diablo Blvd., Lafayette, CA 94549. (800)
227-2334.

Other factors which make you more susceptible to bronchitis
include living and sleeping in damp conditions, exposure to coal dust
and smoke, and low general resistance to infection (see section 5.12).
If you can attend to these problems you can become free from
bronchitis.

5.12 IMPROVING YOUR IMMUNITY TO INFECTION

If you suffer from recurrent infections of any type you need to look at
your total lifestyle. Something in the way you live—perhaps a whole
variety of aspects of your everyday life—is depressing your immune
responses.

Over the course of the last century, excitement about the discovery
of infectious organisms and their role in illness has led us to neglect
the crucial importance of maintaining our general resistance. We
have concentrated too much on the agents of disease and too little on
ourselves, the unwilling hosts. Medicine tries to find more and better
ways of killing germs, while other aspects of our culture make us ever
more susceptible to them. It is a battle that we will lose unless we
look to the way we live.

Think about the relevance to your life of the following points.

1. Recurring or persistent respiratory symptoms may be related to
   allergy rather than to infection (see chapter 6).
2. Good nutrition is essential to a high level of immunity (see chapter
   18, particularly sections 18.2 and 18.4(*a*), (*d*), (*f*), (*h*), (*j*) and (*k*).
3. Pollution is an important source of problems. The chronic load of
   chemical pollution in our food, water and air stresses the immune
   system, forcing it to discriminate between many more substances
   than it was ever designed to do. The more you are able to reduce
   your internal pollution level, the more effective your defenses
   against infection are likely to be. (See sections 18.2, 18.8 and

18.10 for advice on reducing the level of chemical pollution in your diet; sections 6.11 and 6.12 explain how to reduce the pollution level in your environment.)

4. Stress—due to overwork, obsessive exercise, chronic anxiety or any other cause—depresses the immune system and reduces resistance to infection. If you start to suffer frequent infections you should reassess your priorities. Are you trying to do more than is possible for you? Are you taking responsibility for areas of life for which you should not be responsible? Are you failing to give yourself sufficient time to recover from the demands your way of life makes on you? Infections are a form of warning; if you fail to heed them, you may be setting yourself up for more serious physical breakdown.

   Everyone needs rest. You need to sleep until you wake naturally, and you need to have days off. You can push yourself for a little while, but push yourself too long and your health will suffer. Your performance will suffer too; you will spend more and more time achieving less and less. There's no sense in it. (See chapter 16 for advice on reducing your stress level.)

5. Unhappiness and loss also make us vulnerable to infection. Any severe disruption or loss—of status, income, a home or of someone who was dear to us—is stressful and will depress immune functioning. At these times it is more important than ever to look after yourself, to rest enough and eat well. (See section 4.2 if your poor resistance to infection could be linked with depression.)

6. Smoking damages immunity, increasing your susceptibility to infections, allergies and cancers.

6

Respiratory Allergies

This chapter deals with common respiratory problems that are not due to infection. They include seasonal allergies that affect the nose and chest, such as hay fever and allergic asthma, and problems that continue all year round, such as perennial rhinitis (chronic runny nose), breathlessness and asthma.

Respiratory allergies are very common indeed. Surveys suggest that one person in six suffers from hay fever, while one child in ten and one adult in twenty suffers from asthma. These problems are rapidly becoming more common; hay fever did not exist at all before the Industrial Revolution in the nineteenth century, and though asthma has been recognized for thousands of years, the incidence of childhood asthma has risen sixfold in the last thirty years. The prevalence of perennial rhinitis is not known. Asthma is by far the most serious of these conditions, killing more than three thousand people per year.

While many sufferers from respiratory allergies become free of *symptoms during adulthood, increasing numbers of mature people are developing symptoms for the first time. The severity of these conditions typically varies from month to month and from year to year. Sufferers may have no problems at all for long periods. The fluctuations are related to aspects of the sufferer's life and circumstances, and to environmental factors such as the weather.*

SECTION INDEX

6.1   *Allergy: its nature and causes*

6.2   *Hay fever*

6.3   *Perennial rhinitis*

6.4   *Drugs for hay fever and perennial rhinitis*

6.5   *Alternatives to drugs for hay fever*

6.6   *Alternatives to drugs for perennial rhinitis*

6.7   *Asthma and breathlessness*

6.8   *Drugs for asthma*

6.9   *Alternatives to drugs for asthma*

6.10 *Asthma and allergy*

6.11 *Reducing susceptibility to allergic reactions*

6.12 *Dealing with house-dust mite*

6.13 *Reducing environmental pollution*

6.1   ALLERGY: ITS NATURE AND CAUSES

Allergies develop when the immune system overreacts to particular substances. (See sections 5.1 and 5.2.) To protect us from infection, the mast cells which line the respiratory passages assess and identify every particle, substance and organism in the air that enters the body. Unfortunately, twentieth-century life exposes us to so many artificial substances that the mast cells' identification systems are increasingly likely to break down. These systems do not have an unlimited capacity for precise discrimination among such a huge range of substances, and those that are similar to one another easily get confused. Harmless fungal spores can get confused with dangerous forms, and tiny grains of pollen can get confused with invading pathogens, such as bacteria, which may have similar protein coats. Perceiving these harmless substances as serious hazards, the system strives mistakenly to protect us from them, causing the mast cells to flood the area with histamines and an assortment of other substances which are produced to incapacitate pathogens.

When this happens in the upper part of the respiratory system—the nose and throat—we experience many of the same symptoms we suffer when we are under attack from cold viruses. We may feel localized heating, the nose starts to stream with runny mucus, and the membranes become sore and inflamed. The overall effect may be indistinguishable from a cold, but it can continue for very much longer and it is often more severe because the substances which stimulate the reaction are present in much larger quantities and over longer periods than cold viruses.

If the reaction occurs further down the respiratory system, the flood of chemicals—notably histamine—from the bursting mast cells, and the swelling and inflammation induced by the reaction, can close down the bronchial tubes, causing great difficulty in breathing. The effect is asthma.

Asthma and other respiratory symptoms often seem unrelated to allergy, though it is likely that allergy is involved in almost every case. It can be very difficult to identify the substances which trigger the reaction, for while respiratory allergies are most often associated with overreaction to substances in the air, they can also be triggered by substances that enter our bodies in other ways. Sensitivity to particular foods, chemicals, drugs and even (though very rarely) to substances like one's husband's semen, can result in asthmatic attacks or sneezing, sore eyes and runny nose.

In the face of the staggering rise in the incidence of serious environmental illness, the rational answer to these problems must be prevention. We have to rethink some of our priorities and learn to live in a different way. It is often possible to avoid the onset of respiratory allergy, and there are steps that responsible parents should take to prevent their children from developing these conditions. Some of these are described in sections 6.10 and 6.11, while sections 15.1 to 15.3 give more information for potential parents.

6.2   HAY FEVER

Hay fever is characterized by a combination of respiratory symptoms: sneezing, runny nose, sore eyes and throat, and itchy ears and mouth. It is seasonal, developing at any time from about March to July, and it lasts from a few hours or days to several months. The timing corresponds with the concentration in the air of particular pollens or spores to which the sufferer has become sensitive.

The peak season for hay fever is June to August, when ragweed and grasses are in flower; ragweed pollen is the most common hay fever trigger in the United States. Tree pollens can trigger hay fever from early spring, and mold spores add their contribution from about July to October. The hay fever season begins earlier in Southern states, but the majority of sufferers are in the industrial Northeast.

6.3   PERENNIAL RHINITIS

Symptoms similar to those of a cold or hay fever that last throughout the year are due to perennial rhinitis. This is usually caused by allergy to house-dust mite (see section 6.12), though sufferers may be allergic to a range of other substances in their everyday environment. Treatment is generally similar to that for hay fever.

6.4   DRUGS FOR HAY FEVER AND PERENNIAL RHINITIS

(a) Antihistamine

Many medicines containing antihistamines are available without a prescription. Products for allergy include: Actidil, Actifed, Afrin, Afrinol, Allerest, Benadryl, Chlor-Trimeton, Comtrex, Corcidin, Delacort, Demazin, Dimetane, Dimetapp, Disophrol, Dristan, Drixoral, Fedahist, Nostril, Nostrilla, Novahistine, Pyrroxate, Ryna Liquid, Sinarest, Sudafed, Teldrin, Triaminic, Vicks Sinex Decongestant.

Antihistamines counter some of the more unpleasant effects of the histamine which is released from bursting mast cells. They will stop your nose running but most forms are likely to make you feel drowsy. You should not drive or operate machinery when taking them, as you are much more likely to have an accident. Alcohol exaggerates the effect of antihistamines on the brain. A new drug, terfenadine (Seldane), is said by the manufacturers not to produce drowsiness. It is available by prescription only.

Antihistamines have other side effects, including an assortment of effects on the brain and nervous system. They can affect mood, appetite and activity level, and they can cause weight gain, stomach problems, blurred vision, dry mouth and perceptual changes. Some people can become allergic to medications that contain antihistamine.

A disturbing possibility is that by blocking the body's defense systems, antihistamines may make users more susceptible to infection. Such an effect would be difficult to detect and would not be discovered through conventional animal experiments used in drug safety tests.

(b) Cromolyn Sodium

Cromolyn Sodium (Intal, Nasalcrom, Opticrom) is a drug which is used to coat the surface of the mast cells so that they do not react to allergens such as pollen. You can use it before your hay fever begins, and continue to use it regularly to avoid the symptoms, but it is not meant for use once the allergic reaction has begun because it will not suppress it. As with antihistamines, the effects of these products on the body's resistance to infection is a matter for conjecture; we find it hard to believe that blocking a defense system will not increase the possibility of infection.

(c) Decongestant sprays and nose drops

The following products contain decongestant drugs: Afrin Nasal Spray, Benzedrex Inhaler, Coricidin Decongestant Nasal Mist, Dristal, Duration 12 Hour Nasal Spray, 4-Way Nasal Spray, NT2, Neo-

Synephrine, Nostril Nasal Decongestant, Otrivin, Privine and Vicks Sinex.

Decongestant drugs are discussed in section 5.5. They are particularly hazardous for people with heart and blood-pressure problems, though healthy people are sometimes sensitive to them.

Decongestant sprays and drops have additional side effects of their own. They can irritate the nose and cause headaches and palpitations. If you use them for long periods (how long will vary between individuals) you will become dependent on them; when you cease to use them you will suffer "rebound congestion" and your nose will become blocked. The damage to the nose may be long-lasting and even permanent.

(d) Steroids

Steroids (strictly, corticosteroids) are synthetic forms of hormones produced by the adrenal gland of the body. They reduce inflammation and other symptoms of allergic reactions. Steroid preparations can be sprayed directly onto body membranes, used on the skin, taken in tablet form or given by injection.

There are many types and many forms; the list of brand names given below is far from complete and not all the products in the list are used for all the numerous conditions that are treated with steroids.

Steroid brand names

Beclomethasone dipropionate (Beclovent Inhaler, Beconase Inhaler and Nasal Spray, Vancenase Inhaler, Vanceril Inhaler); betamethasone (Celestone); cortisone acetate (Cortone); dexamethasone (Aeroseb-Dex, Daladone, Decadron, Decaspray, Dexasone, Hexadrol); hydrocortisone (A-hydroCort, Hydrocortone); methylprednisolone (A-methaPred, Depo-Medrol, Depo-Predate, Medrol); prednisolone (Hydeltrasol, Predate 50, Prediapred, Prelone); prednisone (Deltasone, Liquid Pred Syrup, Prednicen-M, Sterapred); triamcinolone (Aristocort, Cinomide, Cyklokapron, Kenalog).

Steroids are very powerful drugs. They can save lives and they can kill and maim. They are very effective in suppressing allergic and inflammatory reactions, but regular use of steroids is extremely risky unless the dose is kept very low. Tablets and injections are more dangerous than sprays.

Corticosteroid hormones are essential to normal healing and recovery systems. The body produces large quantities at times of physiological stress—for example, when you suffer injury or infection. If you take corticosteroids as medicines, this will tend to suppress the body's natural production, so you may not be capable of producing sufficient steroid hormones when they are required to meet urgent need. People who have taken steroids for months or years at a time become incapable of surviving without them, and the prospect for such individuals of a lifetime of dependence on steroids is bleak indeed.

Steroids can stunt the growth of children. Steroid-dependent people suffer a wide range of metabolic problems, from weakening of the bones (resulting in spontaneous fractures) to diabetes and heart disease. Their bodies become bloated while their limbs shrivel. They become highly susceptible to infection.

Most allergists warn against the use of steroids (except for sprays) for hay fever, but some doctors seem still to be unaware of the seriousness of their hazards.

(e) Immunotherapy

Allergy sufferers are sometimes offered a course of injections containing small amounts of the substance to which they are allergic. While some experts believe that this is a good way of reducing the body's overreaction to allergens, it is an unreliable procedure. Many people fail to benefit, some get worse, and some die. It is impossible to predict what the result will be.

Immunotherapy (also known as desensitization) is far more popular in the United States than in Britain. It may be a useful remedy for some sufferers when given by specialized allergists who take all the necessary precautions. If you are considering this course of action, *make sure you stay on the doctor's premises for an hour after each injection; ensure that oxygen and epinephrine are available in case you should suffer a reaction, and report any illness (including itching and especially breathlessness) immediately.*

6.5 ALTERNATIVES TO DRUGS FOR HAY FEVER

Although hay fever is triggered by pollens, the underlying cause is general immune-system overload. Reduce your susceptibility to allergy by following the advice given in sections 6.11, 6.12 and 6.13. Take action before the season starts in order to improve your chances of staying free from hay fever.

If your symptoms begin early in the year—from late February to early May—you are probably reacting to tree pollens. Try to identify the source of your problem. Pollen from trees will float in the air over large distances, though it will be concentrated near the trees. Avoid them when they are in flower. If you are moving, don't choose a new home that is close to trees that affect you.

Symptoms in June and July are likely to be related to ragweed pollen. This bright yellow daisylike flower grows on cultivated and waste ground in many parts of the United States. Symptoms from April in Southern states to August in Northern states are usually triggered by grass pollens. Some people react to pollens from other weeds such as nettles.

It is difficult to avoid grass or ragwort pollen but you can reduce your exposure by staying indoors with windows and doors closed in the afternoons, especially on bright sunny days when your symptoms are likely to be at their worst. You're likely to be safest after rain—especially fine drizzly rain, which clears the air. Don't go camping in fields containing your allergy trigger. If you react to grass pollen, don't lie on the grass or mow the lawn. If you can take a holiday in a beach resort in a different part of the country, you're likely to find that your symptoms disappear.

Again, you should try to find out what you react to and avoid it if you can. You may find that your symptoms get much worse after visits to particular places. Keep a detailed diary so that you find out as much as possible about your particular problem. If you can avoid the places or situations that lead to the exacerbation of your symptoms, you will be able to keep your allergy under control for more of the time.

Showy garden flowers and houseplants are not likely to cause you any ill effects, so you need not throw them out. It is important to remove any synthetic sources of perfumes, but you need not worry about most natural ones.

6.6   ALTERNATIVES TO DRUGS FOR PERENNIAL RHINITIS

If you suffer from what seems to be perpetual hay fever or a chronic cold, and you sneeze or your nose runs all year round, you are probably allergic to something in your diet or environment. Study sections 6.11, 6.12 and 6.13 for advice on actions you can take to eliminate or at least minimize the problem.

Check the times when your symptoms are worst and see if you can relate them to the environmental factors. For example, a nose problem and stuffiness that are worst when you wake in the morning or when you are lying in bed are likely to be related to house-dust mite and/or feather bedding or pillows (see section 6.12). If your problem is with you wherever you are, at all times, it may be associated with a food allergy. Dairy produce is a common cause.

Perennial rhinitis can also be caused by treatment with nasal sprays. The only thing you can do if this is the case is to stop treating your runny nose; with luck the membranes will recover. Eat plenty of foods rich in vitamins C and E (see sections 18.4(f) and (h)) to aid healing.

6.7   ASTHMA AND BREATHLESSNESS

In an asthma attack the mast cells lining the tubes to the lungs burst open, causing inflammation and swelling which partially blocks the airways. Breathing out becomes particularly difficult, and carbon dioxide builds up in the overinflated lungs. As the attack progresses the sufferer begins to cough. Lack of air causes restlessness and anxiety and the skin develops a blue tinge. Usually the attack will abate after a while, but there is tremendous variation among asthmatics and among attacks.

Asthma can be fatal, and severe acute asthma which continues unabated for more than half an hour despite the use of inhalers is likely to require hospital treatment. This is especially important if the pulse rate is high (usually over 110 beats per minute) and the sufferer is blue, restless and exhausted. If this is the case you must call a doctor. If you can't get a doctor *immediately*, take the asthmatic to the nearest hospital.

While most asthma is related to allergy (see section 6.10), it can sometimes be a symptom of heart problems. Breathlessness accompanied by pain in the chest can be a symptom of hyperventilation; this is more common among mature people than among children (see section 16.12 for advice).

6.8 DRUGS FOR ASTHMA

Three major types of drugs are prescribed for asthmatics:

(a) Cromolyn Sodium

Cromolyn Sodium (Intal) protects sufferers from allergic asthma. It is a very safe drug and can completely prevent asthma attacks, but it does not work for all asthmatics and is of no benefit once an attack has started.

(b) Bronchodilators

Bronchodilators open up the bronchial tubes. These drugs fall into two subgroups: epinephrine and related drugs, and theophylline derivatives. Some products, including Marax, Mudrane GG Elixir, Primatene Tablets (M and P Formulas), Tedral and Theofedral Tablets, contain both types of drug. Some contain other ingredients such as caffeine, antihistamines and atropine. Reference books such as the *Physicians' Desk Reference* give complete lists of ingredients in these products.

Products containing epinephrine include: Ayerst Epitrate, Broncholate, EpiPen, Marax, Medihaler-Epi, Mudrane Tablets, Primatene, Quadrinal Tablets, Quelidrine Syrup, Rynatuss, Tedral Elixir and Tablets, Theofedral, Vaponefrin. Epinephrine is related to the decongestants described in section 5.5 and has similar side effects. Some of the drugs that contain it can stimulate the heart, causing rapid beating, chest pain and heartbeat irregularities, so people with heart problems should avoid them. Overuse of pressurized aerosols related to some members of this group has killed thousands of asthmatics. Never use these products more often than advised on the pack; do not use them more than once an hour.

Products containing theophylline and its derivatives, the second group of bronchodilators, include: Accurbron, Aerolate, Aminophylline, Aquaphyllin, Asbron, Bronkodyl, Constant-T, Duraphyl, Elixophyllin, Marax, Mudrane GG, Primatene Tablets, Quadrinal, Respbid, Slo-bid, Slo-Phyllin, Somophyllin, Sustaire, Tedral, Theo-24, Theobid, Theochron, Theoclear, Theo-Dur, Theofedral, Theolair, Theon, Theo-Organidin, Theospan-SR, Theostat, Theovent, Uniphyl. These drugs relax bronchial muscles, stimulate the respiratory center of the brain and increase the blood supply to the heart. Side effects include stomach irritation, nausea and vomiting. Never take these tablets with coffee, but if you are caught without your asthma tablets, try drinking a couple of cups of strong coffee instead.

(c) Steroids

Steroids are used for severe asthma. They may be given by injection, in tablet form or in inhalers. Section 6.4(d) includes some steroid brand names and describes their side effects.

The hazards of steroids are balanced by the seriousness of asthma. Inhalers are less hazardous than tablets and injections because the dose is smaller and it is believed that most of it is not absorbed into the system. Nevertheless, the dangers of steroid inhalers should not be underestimated. They may provide good relief from asthma but at the unavoidable cost of decreased resistance to infection, especially fungus infection of the mouth and throat, and damage to the membranes onto which the drug is sprayed. The adverse effects of steroid tablets are likely to be shared by inhalers although they will be less severe and will develop more slowly.

6.9 ALTERNATIVES TO DRUGS FOR ASTHMA

To reduce the severity and frequency of asthma attacks, you may have to take action in every area of your life. For most asthmatics the triggers are numerous and it is rarely possible to eliminate all of them. However, there is much you can do to minimize the problem.

(a) Breathing

Many asthmatics develop a breathing pattern which is rapid and shallow and which uses the upper chest and shoulders. This can make each attack more serious and reduces the control you have over the problem. You should learn "abdominal breathing"—a slow, deep way of breathing like a sleeping baby.

The best way to develop breath control and strengthen your abdominal breathing muscles is to take singing lessons with a trained and competent teacher. If you can't imagine yourself singing, take up a wind instrument such as the clarinet, flute, oboe, saxophone, trumpet or tuba; there's a range big enough to suit every musical taste. Again, you will need a good teacher, but the rewards for the asthmatic are tremendous. It does not matter if you think you are never going to be very good at it, or if you think you have a hopeless ear; you will find you get great pleasure out of creating music, and your asthma could improve dramatically. You are more likely to continue working on your breathing if your primary aim is to learn to play your flute like James Galway; reducing the severity of your asthma attacks will become a secondary advantage.

You can also do breathing exercises on your own, without taking music lessons. Lie on your back, with one hand on your upper chest and the other on your stomach. Inhale, breathing in through the nose, counting slowly to two. If you are breathing correctly you will feel your stomach rising. Exhale through your mouth to the count of four with your lips pursed as though slowly inflating a balloon. Repeat as often as you can.

When you are used to abdominal breathing and your tummy—not your upper chest—rises with each breath, you will be able to practice in a variety of positions—sitting, standing, walking or reclining. Put your hand on your abdomen at intervals to check that it is rising and falling correctly. When you are good at abdominal breathing, practice doing it lying down with a weight on your stomach. Start with five pounds (one bag of sugar) and, with your breathing alone, raise and lower the weight. As you get used to lifting these light weights, increase the weight very gradually until you can shift twenty pounds with the power of your chest and diaphragm muscles.

(b) Drainage

Breathing problems can be exacerbated by the accumulation of sticky mucus in the lungs and bronchial tubes. Drink plenty of water to keep the mucus runny so that it will come out. The following exercises should help with this problem, though you would be well advised to consult your doctor or physical therapist on the drainage methods that are most suitable for you.

For these exercises you will need a helper and an inclined bed or bench with one end eighteen inches higher than the other. Use pillows for comfort. Lie down so that your feet are on the higher end and ask your helper to clap your lower ribs with an open hand (like smacking someone on the back to dislodge food that has gone down the wrong way). The helper should do it first on one side of the chest, then on the other, to encourage coughing. Then turn around and lie on your back with your head at the higher end. The helper should then clap your pectoral muscles just in front of the armpits. Then, again lying on the back, but with the feet higher than the head, turn slightly onto one side, supported with pillows. Get your helper to clap the area just above the nipple. Turn on to the other side and repeat.

(c) Exercise

Many asthmatics avoid exercise because they find that it can bring on an attack. However, the correct type of exercise will prove very beneficial, though it is essential that you take precautions. The key is moderation; always stop short of precipitating an attack. The more you do at this level, the more you will be able to do without suffering an attack, and the more your health will benefit.

In general, short periods of one to two minutes of rapid activity followed by rest are most suitable for asthmatics, since continuous strenuous activity such as running is liable to bring on an attack. Stop–start games such as badminton can be fine, and activities such as cycling, where you can alternate between effort and rest, are also good. Swimming and walking are both excellent, and so long as you keep warm, neither is likely to cause problems. Brisk walking should be combined with deep abdominal breathing in unpolluted air for maximum benefit. However, it is essential to protect yourself from cold air; never exercise outside in cold weather, and use a scarf over your nose and mouth to protect yourself whenever you go outside in cold weather.

(d) Relaxation

An asthma attack is a very frightening experience, and fear adds to its severity because it makes breathing problems even worse. It will prove helpful if you can learn to control your anxiety reactions. If at the same time you can also reduce your general level of emotional stress, your attacks are likely to be less frequent. It used to be believed not merely that anxious people were more susceptible to asthma but that the condition was entirely emotional in origin. In fact it is most unlikely that emotional stress alone is capable of causing asthma, though it may cause hyperventilation (see section 16.12), which can trigger asthma attacks in some people.

Learning yoga—not just the exercise part of it but the meditation methods and breathing techniques as well—is a good way to learn conscious relaxation. (See chapter 16 for other techniques.)

Vacations are often extremely helpful for asthmatics. If you can go somewhere where the air is pure and fresh and where you can relax you are sure to benefit. Go to the mountains in the summer if you can; the Swiss sanatoriums made their reputation on the basis of the real advantages of Alpine air for people with breathing problems.

Some spas also specialize in helping people with asthma. Ask a good travel agent for advice.

Finally, you should do all you can to avoid exposure to infections such as colds and to build up your resistance to them (see section 5.12), because infection causes particularly severe problems for people with respiratory allergies.

6.10 ASTHMA AND ALLERGY

In the majority of cases asthma is due to allergy. This is almost always true of children. It is therefore particularly important that you do all you can to identify and avoid everything to which you are allergic and everything which could make you more susceptible to allergy.

Allergic asthma usually begins within minutes of exposure and peaks within half an hour, so check carefully to discover what you might have inhaled shortly before the attack began. Domestic animals—dogs, cats, gerbils, birds—are common triggers. Cat fur is perhaps the worst. Tragically, it is often the asthmatic's own pet to which he or she is most sensitive.

Seasonal asthma is usually worst in late summer, and it is often due to mold spores. The problem is likely to be particularly bad in damp years or when the weather gets warmer after a long spell of rain. The source may be mildew growing on grain in local fields, or molds on almost any organic matter such as rotting window frames or old plaster on walls. You may be forced to move in order to avoid your trigger—an extreme remedy perhaps, but when severe asthma is regularly associated with one's own home, extreme action is called for. It could be enough to cure the problem completely.

Asthma attacks are more common at night, and if this is your experience it would make sense to look for your trigger in the bedroom. Feather pillows and bedding could be the cause, or fungal spores released from the plaster or other parts of the structure of the room when your breathing makes the air sufficiently damp. If your attacks occur regularly at night, try sleeping in another house for a while. See if the pattern of your illness changes, and search for clues to your trigger in your changing susceptibility.

Strong smells of any sort—even cooking odors and perfumes—

can set off allergic reactions in sensitive people. Substances such as paint, solvents, adhesives and other chemicals frequently trigger asthma attacks. Problems are particularly likely to arise in industries concerned with plastics, paint, adhesives and detergents. Because cereal and animal dust and molds can cause allergic lung diseases and asthma, you should be wary of laboratories, farms and baking, brewing or cereal-milling factories.

If the onset of your asthma was related to a change in your working environment, you will seriously have to consider changing your job. Your health is likely to go steadily downhill if you continue to be exposed to substances to which you are allergic. Farmer's lung, for example, a condition associated with allergy to cereal dust, eventually kills a substantial proportion of sufferers who fail to change their occupations.

Asthma can result from allergic reactions to foods, chemicals in food, or drugs. One in five asthmatics are sensitive to aspirin—aspirin and related medicines can trigger attacks—so it might be wise to avoid it entirely. Read the labels on other medicines, especially pain and arthritis products and cough or cold remedies (see the lists in sections 5.3, 5.5 and 12.10, but do not assume they are complete) to be sure you are not taking aspirin or ibuprofen or drugs such as salicylate which are related to aspirin. Ask your pharmacist if you are in any doubt. Certain other drugs, notably beta blockers (section 9.3(a)), can also trigger asthma. If your problem began or became much worse when you started a course of drug therapy, ask your doctor about discontinuing or changing the drug.

Some food additives are common asthma triggers, and may make the problem worse for people who are already reacting to other allergens (see section 18.10 for details).

Two further points about food. It is unwise for an asthma sufferer to eat a very large meal since this can put pressure on the diaphragm and precipitate an attack. Also, avoid having meals just before going to bed.

Minimizing the risk of allergy in children

Parents and parents-to-be who want to minimize the risk that their children will develop allergies should do all they can to avoid pollutants and other substances which add to their own allergic loading. Following the general recommendations in this chapter on diet and environment will help. It is particularly important that pregnant women avoid polluting their bodies with potentially harmful chemicals from the food they eat and the air they breathe.

6.11   REDUCING SUSCEPTIBILITY TO ALLERGIC REACTIONS

The best way of tackling any allergy is to tackle its causes by reducing the stress on the immune system. An analogy developed by the Norwegian health services may help you to understand the strategy. Think of the capacity of your immune system to deal with potential allergens as a bucket. Some people have larger buckets than others, and they can tolerate higher levels of allergens. Symptoms develop when your system is exposed to more than it can handle and the bucket overflows. The way to deal with the problem is to empty the bucket by reducing the level of potentially allergenic substances that you meet in everyday life.

Cutting the total load of chemicals to which you are exposed will reduce your susceptibility. You should also try to identify specific substances to which you are allergic by keeping a careful record of your symptoms and their fluctuations in relation to the time of day and where you are so that you can reduce your exposure to them.

Most asthmatics and hay fever sufferers actually have multiple allergies. To make matters worse, once you start reacting to one substance you become more susceptible to other potential allergens in your environment. Hay fever sufferers may react to a range of grass pollens, tree pollens, mold spores and house-dust mite—but only during their hay fever season. They may have no symptoms at all outside the season even if some of these allergens are present in their environment.

Food allergies are increasingly common and can cause respiratory symptoms which usually begin ten to fifteen minutes after eating the problem food, though symptoms can be delayed by some hours. (See section 18.8 for more information.) Although you may not be aware of any specific food allergies, you can reduce your general allergy problem by making sure you have a healthy diet with the minimum quantity of chemical pollutants. This means eating simple, unprocessed foods, preferably organically grown (see section 18.2). Essential fatty acids (see section 18.4(*o*)) are particularly important for protection from allergy. Make sure your diet contains plenty of unprocessed vegetable fats, seeds and fish, and cut your intake of margarine and other processed vegetable-oil products. Refuse white bread unless you know it is free from chemicals, avoid "junk" and processed food, and read labels assiduously so that you do not consume additives unknowingly. Steer clear of products such as factory-made soups and desserts, soft drinks and candy, and anything with an unnaturally bright color. These types of food are in reality chemical cocktails that will exacerbate allergic susceptibility.

6.12 DEALING WITH HOUSE-DUST MITE

Whether your problem is asthma, hay fever, a perpetually runny nose or a chronically blocked-up head, you are likely to react badly to house-dust mites. The ubiquitous mite is the most common allergen in the world.

Dust mites are tiny creatures that live on the flakes of skin that we shed continually as we sleep and when we change our clothes. The highest level of mites is found in the bedroom—in your bedding, in your pillows, in your teddy bear, on the floor, in the dust on the dresser—everywhere. When you lie in bed your nose is particularly close to high concentrations of them.

How much trouble you are willing to take obviously depends on the severity of your illness. Asthmatics may be more willing to change their living environment than those hay fever sufferers who are troubled by their allergy for only a few weeks in a bad year. Ideally, all allergy sufferers should sleep in a Norwegian-style bedroom, with varnished or painted wood and rugs which can be washed regularly rather than thick-pile fitted carpets.

The bed is particularly important; on average it contains about 10,000 mites! Choose bedding made from synthetic fibers that can go through the washing machine weekly if possible. Do not use biological detergents in the wash because they are often linked with allergy; a safe washing powder is Ecover, available from health-food stores. Avoid bedding or pillows containing feathers or down. Wash your pillows monthly. Don't take toys or stuffed animals to bed. Cover your mattress completely with a plastic sheet so that mites don't build up in it. Foam mattresses are less attractive to mites than interior-spring types.

Vacuum cleaning is very helpful, though the allergy sufferer should try to get someone else to do it. Clean thoroughly and frequently around and under the bed, and vacuum the mattress when changing the sheets. Always get someone else to empty the vacuum cleaner. Use a damp mop or cloth to keep all surfaces free of dust.

Mites thrive in warm, dark, damp conditions. Keeping the bedroom well aired, hanging bedding in the sun and avoiding heaters that produce water vapor will help keep their numbers down.

6.13 REDUCING ENVIRONMENTAL POLLUTION

Air pollution is a serious hazard for those who suffer from respiratory problems. Try to avoid breathing air that is polluted by smoke, chemicals or fumes. Smoking—whether by you or those close to you—will undoubtedly make your problem worse. Avoid sprays of all kinds; never use fly killers or air fresheners, hair spray or any other aerosol product. Pesticides (including those you use on your house plants) are particularly likely to add to your problems.

Cleaning products, especially heavy duty detergents, are very common allergens. Use the simplest products you can even if you don't get such a bright wash; pure soap is least likely to affect you. Look for products in the Ecover range. Avoid any products that leave a "fresh" perfume on your clothes or furniture; that smell will in reality be yet another chemical pollutant that could add to your allergy problem.

An ionizer may reduce your allergic problems. Some people are convinced that they experience real benefit from using one, though there is conflicting evidence on this. It will at least do no harm, and many of the companies which sell ionizers offer a money-back guarantee, so you can try their products for a couple of months without committing yourself.

Photochemical smog, such as that which hovers over Los Angeles, contains pollutants that are very dangerous to asthmatics; it will make all respiratory allergies worse. Living or working in this sort of atmosphere may seriously damage the health of people who are vulnerable to it. If your allergy problems are severe, you may have to consider staying (or moving) away from these areas.

7

Skin Disorders

This chapter deals with acne and other spots and rashes; allergic skin disorders including eczema, urticaria, angioedema, dermatitis and psoriasis; fungal and bacterial infections; and leg ulcers.

SECTION INDEX

7.1 The skin: what it is and how it works
7.2 Pimples and acne
7.3 Drugs for acne
7.4 Alternatives to drugs for pimples and acne
7.5 Rashes and dermatitis
7.6 Drugs for rashes and dermatitis
7.7 Alternatives to drugs for rashes and dermatitis
7.8 Urticaria and angioedema
7.9 Drugs for urticaria and angioedema
7.10 Alternatives to drugs for urticaria and angioedema

7.11 *Eczema*

7.12 *Drugs for eczema*

7.13 *Alternatives to drugs for eczema*

7.14 *Psoriasis*

7.15 *Drugs for psoriasis*

7.16 *Alternatives to drugs for psoriasis*

7.17 *Skin infections*

7.18 *Drugs for skin infections*

7.19 *Alternatives to drugs for skin infections*

7.20 *Leg ulcers*

7.1 THE SKIN: WHAT IT IS AND HOW IT WORKS

The skin is the largest of the body's organs. It cools us down or conserves heat; it shields us from external hazards and helps to eliminate internal ones; it houses our sense of touch; and it gives out signals to others about our mood and state of health.

The surface of the skin is dead, the cells being filled with a tough protein called keratin which protects the vulnerable living cells beneath. The surface layer keeps out most of the substances with which we come into contact, but substances that are capable of dissolving oils can penetrate it. Few such substances existed in the natural environment in which our ancestors evolved, so the skin has few defenses against them.

The skin is lubricated by a special oil called sebum which is secreted by sebaceous glands just below the surface. This forms an additional waterproofing layer, but it is readily removed by washing with detergents and soaps, so it tends to be kept to a minimum by most people in our excessively hygiene-conscious society.

Sweat glands are found over the whole surface of the skin. These are important for temperature regulation, and perhaps more importantly for most of us, they are also part of a chemical signaling system which transmits subtle messages to others by creating our own individual smell. This varies from time to time according to hormone changes and stress. The "smell of fear," for example, is far more than just a cliché; it is a detectable reality. Similarly, our sweat can transmit the smell of sexual arousal, produced by the pheromones, that attract people of the opposite (or the same) sex.

The sebum and sweat glands also act as organs of excretion. Their products may contain residues of food we have eaten, of chemicals we have absorbed or waste from metabolic processes. Hence the smell of alcohol, garlic, drugs or chemicals can linger on our bodies until they are completely excreted and washed away. These natural secretions are mildly antibiotic; healthy, intact skin is capable of combating the bombardment of potentially infective organisms to which we are constantly exposed. Because these secretions form an important protective layer, you should try not to wash them off too often. Far more problems are caused by excessive washing than by lack of hygiene. Soaps containing deodorants are unnecessary, and bathing in disinfectants is foolish. The best form of skin care involves minimal interference with the natural balance of the skin; the simplest soaps are least likely to cause harm.

7.2 PIMPLES AND ACNE

Temporary blemishes on the skin are usually related to the skin's eliminatory function. They are, in a nutshell, a reaction to pollution, whether it be by infection, chemicals, substances to which one is sensitive, or breakdown products of hormones present in excess, for example during adolescence or early pregnancy. Because these are all processed by the same systems, the skin is particularly likely to react to one substance if it is already overburdened with others.

The majority of adolescents suffer from acne. It develops when sex hormones are produced at a high rate, and it seems to be related to overload of the metabolic processes which break down hormones and environmental chemicals. The sebaceous glands get clogged with these waste products of metabolism and can become infected.

7.3 DRUGS FOR ACNE

These take two general forms: substances applied directly to the skin, particularly cleansing, abrasive and antiseptic products, and drugs taken internally, particularly the antibiotic tetracycline (occasionally also erythromycin or co-trimoxazole). Vitamin A derivatives such as tretinoin (Retin-A) are sometimes used though they can cause skin peeling and excessive sensitivity to sunlight. Tetracycline and other antibiotics are discussed in section 5.7.

Antibiotics for acne are usually prescribed in low doses for between three months and two years. Disadvantages of prolonged antibiotic treatment include damage to the normal function of the gut and the development of hypersensitivity. You may find that if you have been taking tetracycline for some time it will no longer control acute infection because your gut flora have developed resistance to it. This resistance can be transferred from gut bacteria to dangerous pathogens.

Synthetic hormones such as Diane are sometimes prescribed for women with severe acne. These drugs, like oral contraceptives which can also combat acne in some women, may cause thrombosis and cardiovascular problems.

Creams containing steroids and/or antibiotics, such as Cort-Dome, Cortisporin, Cortril, Hydrocortisone cream, Neosporin, Topicycline or Vanoxide-HC Acne Lotion, should be avoided. If you use any cream or lotion for acne, check with your pharmacist to make sure it contains neither antibiotics, which can cause sensitization and allergic skin problems, nor steroids, which have many adverse effects (see sections 6.4(d) and 7.6)—including increased vulnerability to infection.

7.4 ALTERNATIVES TO DRUGS FOR PIMPLES AND ACNE

Part of the treatment strategy for acne and similar problems should be an attempt to rebalance the body's hormone systems. (Women should consult sections 14.1 and 14.4) Sex will help to clear the skin of pimples; sexual frustration will make the problem worse.

Avoid all substances which load the metabolic systems that break down hormones (see section 11.4 for advice). Certain foods, particularly chocolate, sugar, "junk" and fast food, milk products and animal fats may make you break out in pimples. Eat plenty of organic whole foods (see section 18.2), especially those that are rich in zinc and vitamin A (see sections 18.4(a), 18.4(j) and 18.7).

Keeping the skin very clean may reduce the problem of clogged sebaceous glands. Try a face mask of natural oatmeal and warm water mixed to a paste and smeared on the skin; leave it to dry and then rinse off. Many commercially produced face masks are available; if you want to try one, look for the simplest nongreasy product.

Avoid skin creams of all sorts, especially those that are said to kill bacteria. They can cause additional problems through hypersensitivity, and greasy creams will increase the chances of your pores becoming blocked.

A period of high stress, such as exam time, can be relied upon to give the acne sufferer a new crop of pimples. Emotional stress loads the detoxification systems with stress hormones and thus makes the skin more susceptible to problems. In addition, stress hormones may make the skin look yellowish and produce dark circles around the eyes. Reduce the level of stress hormones in your body by getting as much sleep as you want, following the advice in chapter 16 and taking fairly strenuous exercise as often as possible—ideally for half an hour each day. Both your performance and your skin will benefit.

Increasing your activity level will make your skin look healthier and give your hair more shine because the flush that strenuous activity induces brings oxygenated, nutrient-rich blood to the skin in larger quantities. It will also keep the cleansing systems of your body working at peak efficiency. If you need to use rouge to avoid looking like a corpse you are probably getting far too little physical activity. Choose activities that make you sweat (see sections 17.4, 17.7 and 17.9).

Cigarette smoking is damaging to the skin in many ways. Not only do the poisons in the smoke (of which there are more than 200 identified forms) load your detoxification systems, but the reduced oxygen in your blood means that your skin is not so well fed with life-giving oxygen. In addition, smoking robs your body of vitamins. Smokers have skin that ages markedly faster than nonsmokers', so give it up!

7.5 RASHES AND DERMATITIS

Skin rashes are a common reaction to substances the body regards as dangerous. They are the most frequently reported adverse drug reaction, and can vary from a crop of small itchy pimples which disappears quite quickly to a very severe, painful and dangerous reaction akin to extensive burns. A rash after taking a drug such as penicillin is a warning that you are sensitive to it and you should *never* take it again; next time you could have a life-threatening reaction.

However, the situation is not usually so serious. If you develop a rash after inhaling certain solvents it does not mean that you are going to die if you have the misfortune to inhale them again. But you should acknowledge that they put a severe strain on your detoxification systems, that they could make you ill and that they are likely to reduce your tolerance to other chemicals.

Most rashes affect the face and upper trunk. Dermatitis means inflamed skin; while it can appear anywhere it most often affects the hands. A localized rash could be a *contact dermatitis*—a reaction to something that has been absorbed through the skin. There are many possible culprits, from the metal in clothes fasteners or detergent residues left on your clothes after washing, to creams and chemicals which get on your hands or other parts of the skin surface. Careful detective work should reveal the cause of the problem and allow you to avoid it.

7.6   DRUGS FOR RASHES AND DERMATITIS

Steroid sprays and creams of varying strengths are used for many forms of dermatitis. Many of them also contain fungicides or antibiotics. The mildest types are available over the counter without a prescription; brands include CardeCort, Cortaid, Delacort and Hydrocortisone cream.

More potent products require a prescription. Creams containing the most potent steroids include betamethasone (Betatrex, Diprolene, Diprosone, Lotrisone, Maxivate, Valisone), clobetasol (Temovate), and desonide (DesOwen, Tridesilon). These can cause very serious adverse effects.

Steroids can be very effective but very dangerous; they should never be used for long periods. Steroid creams thin the skin and increase susceptibility to infection. Steroids can be absorbed through the skin and cause many serious adverse reactions (see section 6.4(d)). Never use waterproof dressings or plastic pants over steroid creams. Withdrawal from steroid therapy can cause "rebound" worsening of symptoms.

7.7 ALTERNATIVES TO DRUGS FOR RASHES AND DERMATITIS

Most skin rashes require no treatment at all. Soothing lotions such as calamine can be helpful, but generally the body will heal itself; the fewer chemicals you put on its surface the easier healing may be. Avoid products containing lanolin; this is a frequent cause of skin reactions. Zinc oxide or zinc and castor-oil cream—normally used for babies' bottoms—can be useful for many types of rash because the zinc aids healing.

Excessive attention to cleanliness, far from protecting you from skin problems, is likely to cause them. Detergents, soaps, solvents, degreasers and cleansers, particularly perfumed and deodorant forms of these products, should be avoided. Use gloves if you are cleaning the house—but do be sure to check that you are not sensitive to their linings!

Washing products containing enzymes are particularly likely to cause skin rashes. Avoid them. The safest washing products are those in the Ecover range, available from an increasing number of health shops. Even if you are not aware of unpleasant reactions to detergents, dishwashing liquids and other cleaning products, you can be sure that they are putting a load on your detoxification systems and increasing the risk that you will react to other things in your diet or environment.

7.8 URTICARIA AND ANGIOEDEMA

Urticaria is a type of itchy skin rash, often called nettle rash or *hives*. It is a symptom of allergy, and about 20% of the population suffer an attack at some time in their lives. It is often associated with angioedema, a condition affecting deeper layers of the skin, typically in the lips, tongue and around the eye. Angioedema causes swelling which can be very severe.

Both of these reactions can be provoked by a wide range of foods and chemicals in those who are sensitive to them. It may be difficult to work out the cause because they can occur up to ten days after the problem substance was consumed, though usually the time lag is shorter—sometimes just a matter of hours. Culprits are often foods you may not normally eat, such as strawberries, seafood and peanuts.

7.9 DRUGS FOR URTICARIA AND ANGIOEDEMA

Allergic skin rashes can be treated with antihistamine tablets (see section 6.4(*a*)). It is possible to get antihistamine skin creams— Benadryl Anti-Itch Cream is an example—but these should never be used because they are known to cause hypersensitivity reactions; they could just lead to a worse problem!

7.10 ALTERNATIVES TO DRUGS FOR URTICARIA AND ANGIOEDEMA

These conditions generally clear up fairly quickly of their own ac-cord, but sufferers should try to identify the substances to which they are allergic. Many foods can precipitate attacks in sensitive people; seafood, nuts, peanuts and eggs are common triggers. Food additives, especially synthetic colors and preservatives, are particularly likely to cause these reactions (see sections 18.8 and 18.10).

Urticaria is a common sign of aspirin sensitivity. If you get a rash after taking aspirin, you should also avoid food additives and drugs that are closely related to aspirin, such as ibuprofen (see section 5.3(*c*)), and avoid products such as cough mixtures and cold rem-edies, which contain aspirin or salicylates. Inhaled allergens such as house-dust mite and mold spores can cause chronic or recurrent urticaria. Study sections 6.11, 6.12 and 6.13 for advice on dealing with these problems.

7.11   ECZEMA

Eczema is a very itchy allergic skin rash. Bad eczema makes the skin red, raw, weeping and crusted and it can become infected. It usually runs in families, and may be associated with other allergy problems such as hay fever. It is particularly common in children, often occurring behind the ears and knees, in body creases at the elbows and neck, and on the face, trunk and scalp. Most babies grow out of infantile eczema, but it can persist. Like other allergic conditions, it is growing steadily more common with the increasing pollution of our environment.

7.12   DRUGS FOR ECZEMA

Steroid creams (see section 7.6) are often used for eczema.

7.13   ALTERNATIVES TO DRUGS FOR ECZEMA

Susceptibility to eczema often seems to develop before a baby is born, especially if the mother eats large quantities of foods containing particular allergens. Problem foods include all cow's-milk products, eggs and chicken (especially indoor bred), food colorings and preservatives (see section 18.10) and wheat. If you have a family history of eczema, avoid these foods as much as possible during pregnancy and breastfeeding.

Babies fed on cow's milk are more likely to develop eczema, so you should try to breastfeed exclusively for at least four months if you can. However, prolonged breast-feeding has recently been shown to be associated with an increased risk of eczema, because the pollutants in the mother's diet and environment are concentrated in her milk. The answer is for the mother to be very careful with her own diet, to avoid all "junk" and processed food, dairy products and animal fats. Vegetarian mothers have the least polluted breast milk.

Once eczema has developed you will need to take great care to reduce your child's exposure to allergens and to anything that is liable to cause skin irritation (see sections 6.11, 6.12 and 6.13). Dress your child in soft cotton, and never put wool or nylon next to the skin. Choose loose clothing styles that won't make the child sweaty. Disposable diapers may irritate, as may plastic pants.

Watch your child's diet carefully to pick up foods that precipitate eczema. Eggs and milk are very common culprits, as are many food additives. Tomatoes, nuts, chocolate and seafood may also cause problems. Never let an allergic child eat anything containing synthetic colors or preservatives. A whole-food diet with minimal dairy produce is best (see sections 18.2, 18.8 and 18.10).

Eczema sufferers of any age must be especially careful with soaps and cleaning products. Never use anything perfumed, and if possible avoid using soap on the skin. Skin cleansers derived from oatmeal are safest. Washing in hard water can also exacerbate eczema, so get a water softener if you live in a hard-water area.

Patches of eczema can appear anywhere on the body where there is contact with a substance to which you are allergic. Nickel allergy is particularly common, affecting one in seven young women. It can cause dermatitis on the ears (from earrings), thighs (from metal chairs), hands (from faucets, scissors, rings or handles), feet (from buckles, zippers or shoe eyelets), back, waist, hips or neck (from fasteners on clothes). Many alloys, including stainless steel, contain nickel, and sensitive people can be affected even through cloth. The only effective solution to this problem is to avoid nickel or wear protective layers to prevent the metal from touching your skin.

Many other substances can set up an eczemalike contact dermatitis. Careful observation should alert you to the culprit in your own case. Avoidance of the allergen is the only sensible answer.

7.14   Psoriasis

Psoriasis is the name given to an area of red, raised pustules covered with silvery scales. It can occur on any part of the body, though the knees, elbows and scalp are the most usual sites. Sometimes it clears up spontaneously, but it tends to recur. It is most common at times of hormone imbalance, particularly adolescence, pregnancy and menopause.

7.15   DRUGS FOR PSORIASIS

Creams containing salicylic acid or coal tar (Fototar Cream, Hydrisalic Gel, Whitfield's Ointment) are sometimes used to treat psoriasis, but it is often left untreated as these preparations can cause sensitization and allergic reactions. Steroid preparations (see section 7.6) can cause the development of more serious forms of the condition and according to the *Physicians' Desk Reference,* they should generally be avoided.

7.16   ALTERNATIVES TO DRUGS FOR PSORIASIS

The cause of psoriasis is not known, although it can be triggered by drugs, injury, stress and infections. The drugs most frequently linked with the condition are steroids, tranquilizers, aspirin and codeine.

The association with hormones and drugs suggests that psoriasis is related to problems in metabolizing these substances. Dietary measures which aid detoxification should help, as should the avoidance of chemicals which load the detoxification systems. Follow the dietary recommendations in section 18.2, 18.4(*d*), 18.4(*j*) and 18.5(*a*)). Supplementing the diet with chelated zinc (available from health stores) may help.

Avoid too much exposure to strong sunlight, especially if your skin is fair, because sunburn can progress to psoriasis.

Emotional stress exacerbates psoriasis in 50% of sufferers, so relaxation exercises, increased physical activity and other measures which reduce stress are likely to be helpful. Read chapter 16 for more information.

7.17   SKIN INFECTIONS

(a) Herpes (cold sores)

These are caused by a common virus which is readily transmitted by secretions from cold sores. The characteristic red, blistered rash most often appears on the edge of the lips, on the genital organs and occasionally on the eye where it can cause extreme pain. Once the virus has entered the body it will remain dormant there, flaring up at intervals when resistance drops. (See sections 14.20, 14.21 and 14.22.)

(b) Bacterial infections of the skin

Bacteria can cause local inflammation around splinters or just under the skin around a hair root, forming boils. Impetigo is a fairly common skin infection which mainly affects children. If the problem is severe or very painful, antibiotics (see section 5.7) may be necessary.

Local problems can often be treated without drugs. Use salt water, as hot as you can bear it, to bring boils to a head and soften the skin surface to encourage quicker discharge of pus. If you get a splinter that won't come out readily, soak the area in hot salt water for ten minutes before attempting to remove it with tweezers. A scalpel blade (available from stores which sell art and office supplies) can be sterilized in boiling water and used to make a small cut in the skin, allowing removal of the splinter.

Don't use any creams (except if prescribed for impetigo) or disinfectant, as these interfere with the body's natural defenses. Just soak regularly in hot salt water until all signs of infection are gone. However, if the swelling and soreness spread, or if you feel generally unwell, consult your doctor.

Recurrent boils are a sign that your immune defenses are not working properly. Follow the advice in section 5.12 on increasing resistance to infection. If the problem persists it may be a sign of diabetes; check with your doctor, and take action as described in section 10.4.

(c) Fungal infections of the skin

Fungi are frequent causes of skin rashes, especially in warm, moist areas such as the crotch and between the toes (athlete's foot). Fungal rashes are usually itchy and pink, perhaps with little spots or peeling areas or a pattern of reddish rings with clear centers (ringworm).

7.18   DRUGS FOR SKIN INFECTIONS

Fungal infestations of the skin can be treated with a wide range of products available from pharmacists with or without a prescription. Brand names include Fungizone, Lotrimin Cream, Monistat-Derm, Mycelex Cream and Spectazole Cream.

7.19   ALTERNATIVES TO DRUGS FOR SKIN INFECTIONS

Fungal infestation is often very resistant to the measures you take against it, and you will probably have to use one of the creams described above to get rid of it. Guard against reinfestation by avoiding dampness. Olive oil smeared in a light layer on the skin can combat fungi. If you improve your general health by paying more attention to diet you will increase your resistance to skin infections (see section 18.2).

Avoid tight-fitting underwear, and wear only pure cotton next to the skin. Wear loose clothes so you sweat as little as possible. Open sandals are the best shoes for the prevention of athlete's foot.

7.20   LEG ULCERS

These persistent and unpleasant ulcers are caused by inadequate blood supply to the skin of the legs. Smokers are particularly likely to suffer from this problem, so it is yet another reason for quitting the habit. In the short term, leg ulcers are likely to require medical attention; the long-term answer is to improve the effectiveness of the vascular system by following the advice given in section 9.14.

8

Digestive Problems

This chapter deals with stomach and intestinal troubles—
indigestion, nausea and vomiting, hiatal hernia, peptic and duodenal ulcers—and problems with the large intestine, including
irritable bowel (spastic colon), ulcerative colitis, diverticulitis,
constipation, diarrhea and hemorrhoids.

SECTION INDEX

8.1   The digestive system: a guided tour
8.2   Indigestion and heartburn
8.3   Drugs for indigestion
8.4   Alternatives to drugs for indigestion
8.5   Peptic ulcers
8.6   Drugs for peptic ulcers
8.7   Alternatives to drugs for peptic ulcers
8.8   Nausea and vomiting
8.9   Drugs for nausea and vomiting

8.10   *Alternatives to drugs for nausea and vomiting*
8.11   *Diarrhea*
8.12   *Drugs for diarrhea*
8.13   *Alternatives to drugs for diarrhea*
8.14   *Constipation*
8.15   *Drugs for constipation*
8.16   *Alternatives to drugs for constipation*
8.17   *Spastic colon or irritable bowel syndrome*
8.18   *Drugs for irritable bowel syndrome*
8.19   *Alternatives to drugs for irritable bowel syndrome*
8.20   *Inflammatory bowel disease*
8.21   *Hemorrhoids*
8.22   *Drugs for hemorrhoids*
8.23   *Alternatives to drugs for hemorrhoids*

8.1   THE DIGESTIVE SYSTEM: A GUIDED TOUR

The digestive system starts at the mouth, where food is chewed and the first stage of digestion begins with the thorough mixing of digestive enzymes in saliva with mashed-up food. From here it is moved to the stomach via the esophagus. In the stomach it meets a range of digestive juices in a highly acid solution which breaks the food down further. The food then passes through the duodenum, where digestion continues with the help of bile from the gallbladder, into the twenty-foot-long small intestine which absorbs nutrients through its lining. The small intestine opens into the large intestine, which ascends on the right side of the lower abdomen, crosses the body just above the navel and descends on the left side to open at the anus. In the large intestine water and nutrients are absorbed from the digested food.

The intestine is the home of a range of life forms, many of which are beneficial to us in providing vitamins and aiding absorption of nutrients. These life forms (the digestive flora) live in harmony with our body tissues and each other, maintaining a balanced ecology within the gut. But they require the right conditions, and if conditions are unsuitable—because of drug treatment or inappropriate diet—they can get out of balance. This is particularly likely to happen if you take antibiotics, with tetracycline as one of the worst villains; antibiotics kill harmless and beneficial bacteria as well as the pathogens they are meant to destroy, allowing yeasts to flourish. Some doctors believe that overgrowth of yeast inside the intestine has generalized unpleasant consequences for health; for example, it is believed to be implicated in food allergies.

8.2 INDIGESTION AND HEARTBURN

Indigestion can be a symptom of a range of digestive troubles. Most of us are familiar with it after unwise eating; too much rich food and sometimes an excess of smoking or drinking can cause a temporary inflammation of the stomach lining. This produces discomfort in the upper part of the abdomen, causing belching and nausea. The problem will normally settle down quite quickly of its own accord if you stop eating and just drink water.

Pregnant women and very overweight people are vulnerable to a form of heartburn that results from the return (reflux) of acid from the stomach back up the esophagus. This may be caused by hiatal hernia, a condition where the stomach bulges through the diaphragm; it can be uncomfortable but is not normally serious. If this is your problem the best solution is to eat whole foods (see section 18.2) and take regular exercise (see chapter 17). See section 10.8 if you are overweight. Avoid tight clothing.

Recurrent indigestion can be a symptom of more serious illness. The cause could be an ulcer (a) if the pain goes right through to your back, so that it feels not unlike backache; (b) if it is associated with vomiting blood or passing blood in the stools so that they look black and tarry (iron tablets can make your stools black too, so don't panic about ulcers if you are taking iron); or (c) if it comes as a burning or gnawing pain in the middle of the chest up to three hours after meals and often at around 2 A.M. Consult your doctor if you fit into any of these patterns.

Gallbladder and liver disease cause recurrent indigestion, especially after the consumption of fatty foods (see sections 11.2 and

11.5 for more information). Angina can also mimic recurrent indigestion; it is most likely to occur with exercise or when you are upset (see section 9.2).

If you suffer from recurrent indigestion for more than a few weeks, consult your doctor to check for any serious underlying disease.

8.3   DRUGS FOR INDIGESTION

These reduce the acidity of the stomach and are therefore called antacids. Over-the-counter remedies for indigestion and upset stomach are very widely used; almost every household has at least one such medicine. Popular brands include Alka-Mints, Alka-Seltzer, Eno, Milk of Magnesia, Rolaids and Tums. The cheapest effective product is sodium bicarbonate; take a level teaspoonful dissolved in a glass of warm water.

Repeated use of antacids containing sodium bicarbonate has been linked with kidney stones. They should not be used by people with heart or kidney disease, nor by those who suffer from fluid retention, because they increase the blood sodium level and may cause further fluid retention. Never drink milk if you are taking indigestion remedies; it can cause excessive absorption of calcium, leading to loss of appetite, nausea, vomiting, weakness, abdominal pain, constipation, thirst and kidney damage.

A wide range of antacids is available both with and without a prescription. Most contain aluminum or magnesium salts, sometimes both. Products containing magnesium salts, some of which are also used as laxatives (see section 8.15), may cause diarrhea and excessive absorption of magnesium if used frequently or in large doses. Brands include Aludrox, Haley's M-O, Milk of Magnesia, Mylanta, Simeco, Trisilate and WinGel. Aluminum salts such as kaolin (Donnagel-PG, Parepectolin) cause constipation; in addition, aluminum has been linked with brain degeneration (Alzheimer's disease). Products containing aluminum include Amphojel, Camalox, Gaviscon, Gelusil, Maalox, Mylanta, Nephrox and WinGel. Although antacids are often treated as harmless household remedies, each type has disadvantages. Clearly, regular use of antacids cannot be beneficial to your general health.

8.4   ALTERNATIVES TO DRUGS FOR INDIGESTION

Three main factors are involved in indigestion: eating habits, smoking and stress. Whatever its cause, you can help prevent it by eating a health-promoting diet based on whole foods rather than processed forms (see section 18.2), and avoiding sugar, white flour, whole milk and fried food (see chapter 18). Don't eat too much at each meal, since overloading the stomach means it must work harder, and relax for a little while afterward—don't go rushing around immediately. Always chew your food well; bolting it down can lead to digestive problems if the food is not sufficiently mixed with saliva. Eating too fast is often a sign of emotional stress, which itself can cause indigestion. Read chapter 16 and adopt the stress-reducing measures described there if you think that this may be your problem.

Tea, coffee, alcohol, chocolate and cola drinks induce indigestion in some people. Try going without them for a couple of weeks to see if this solves the problem.

Smoking stimulates the production of gastric juices and can cause severe indigestion. It also reduces the efficiency of the valve at the top of the stomach, allowing gastric juices to flow back into the esophagus and causing pain. Stopping smoking could cure your indigestion in addition to conferring innumerable other health benefits.

Finally, hypoglycemia (low blood sugar) may be the cause. Make sure you do not get too hungry before each meal; eat when you need to rather than putting it off till later. A whole-food diet rich in grains (whole-grain bread, cereals and brown rice) and vegetables, particularly peas and beans, will reduce the fluctuations in your blood sugar level. (See section 10.5.)

8.5   PEPTIC ULCERS

Ulcers are deep sores which form in the first part of the digestive system. Those that occur in the stomach are called gastric ulcers; those in the first part of the small intestine are called duodenal ulcers. The general term is peptic ulcer. Ulcer pain occurs when excess stomach acid irritates the lining of the stomach or duodenum. About 10% of people in developed countries get peptic ulcers at some time in their lives, most often during middle age. For unknown reasons they are particularly likely to flare up in the spring and autumn. If other members of your family have had ulcers you could be prone to them too.

8.6   DRUGS FOR PEPTIC ULCERS

Your doctor may prescribe one or more of a range of drugs of different types. You may be advised to take antacids (see section 8.3) and/or drugs that reduce the production of stomach acid and/or licorice derivatives. Since ulcers are symptoms of stress, your doctor might also offer you a tranquilizing drug (see section 4.6).

Antacids neutralize stomach acid, thus relieving ulcer pain. Unfortunately, the presence of antacid in the stomach stimulates production of acid by the cells in the lining of the stomach, so initial relief may be followed by a flare-up of pain. Antacids do not increase the rate at which ulcers heal.

(a) Drugs that reduce acid production

This group includes atropine (Antrocol, Atrohist LA, Donnagel, Donnatal), belladonna (Belladenal), dicyclomine (Bentyl), propantheline (Pro-Banthine) and scopolamine (Donnagel-PG).

These products contain anticholinergic drugs which affect input to the stomach from the nerves which stimulate it. Their most frequent side effects are due to effects on other parts of the nervous system, and include blurred vision, dry mouth, rapid heartbeat, urine retention and constipation. They should not be taken by those who suffer from glaucoma or heart disease. Antihistamines (see section 6.4(a)) and antipsychotic drugs (section 4.12) can increase the side effects of these drugs.

(b) H₂ blockers

This group of drugs includes cimetidine (Tagamet), famotidine (Pepcid) and ranitidine (Zantac). They are antihistamines (see section

6.4(*a*)), though their effects are uncharacteristic of that class. They inhibit the production of stomach acid and enhance ulcer healing. Adverse reactions include diarrhea, muscle pains, dizziness and occasionally breast enlargement and skin rashes.

8.7 ALTERNATIVES TO DRUGS FOR PEPTIC ULCERS

Peptic ulcers will heal spontaneously if the conditions which generate them are removed. A life-style that enhances your general health will prevent their recurrence.

(*a*) Diet

For many years, ulcer patients were told to keep to a bland diet consisting mainly of milk, eggs, processed cereals and overcooked vegetables. Recently it has been acknowledged that this sort of thoroughly unhealthy diet is actually harmful to ulcer patients, as it would be for anyone else. Regular drinks of milk were recommended because milk often reduces ulcer pain, but since it can stimulate greater secretion of stomach acid it is not as beneficial as it may seem. On balance, whole milk should probably be avoided, as should cheese and other milk derivatives.

Sugar and white flour seem to promote ulcer formation. If you are concerned about your general health you will probably have already decided to give up eating these nonfoods.

Coffee, strong tea, soft drinks and alcohol may also increase ulcer problems. Make your own judgments about these beverages by tuning into their long- as well as short-term effects on your body. You may have fewer episodes of ulcer pain if you change to diluted fruit juice, water or herb teas.

Eat at least three meals a day. You may feel better on five or six small meals, but individual needs vary. Get to know the meal schedule with which your stomach is most comfortable.

Some foods are likely to upset you, particularly curries and hot-peppered or highly spiced dishes. If your ulcer is particularly troublesome within three hours of a meal (less with a gastric ulcer), you may have eaten something to which you react badly. In time you will

discover the foods that you should avoid. Beware, though, of con-
demning wholesome or enjoyable foods when your ulcer may have
flared up for emotional reasons; a stressful lunch is likely to be more
harmful to you than one that includes unsuitable food.

Choose a diet that is rich in fiber, vitamins A and E, and zinc (see
sections 18.3, 18.4(a), 18.4(h) and 18.4(j). Always chew food well
and never hurry your meals. Your food needs to be very thoroughly
mixed with saliva, which contains substances that protect the lining
of the intestine.

(b) Drugs

Certain drugs can accelerate ulcer formation. These include aspirin
and related drugs such as most of those prescribed for arthritis (see
sections 5.3 and 12.10) and steroids (sections 6.4(d), 6.8(c) and
7.6). Avoid all of these if you can. Many other drugs, including
antihistamines (section 6.4(a)), can also irritate the stomach.

(c) Smoking

Peptic ulcers are more common and relapse rates are higher among
smokers. Your smoking may be in response to the stress that is the
underlying cause of your ulcer. In any case, find a more effective and
less damaging way of managing stress.

(d) Stress

Psychologists have discovered that it is possible to induce stomach
ulcers in animals by subjecting them to stress. Just a few hours can be
enough if the stress is sufficiently severe. Similarly intense stress
(such as that caused by extensive burns) can generate ulcers in
humans within days.

Psychological stress induces increased production of stomach acid,
which can inflame the stomach lining. At the same time it reduces
the body's ability to protect and heal itself. If you react to stress by
drinking coffee and/or alcohol, by forgetting to eat or bolting hurried
meals, or by smoking cigarettes, you increase your chances of devel-

oping an ulcer. You probably know what your major stress generators are; your ulcer is a reminder that you must find a better way to deal with them. Something has to change in your life and it will be up to you to set the necessary change in motion. Study chapter 16 for suggestions on stress management, and consider getting expert help from a counselor or therapist who specializes in emotional problems.

8.8   Nausea and vomiting

These are symptoms which can occur with many kinds of physical or psychological disorders. Some disorders are short-lived, such as mild food poisoning or witnessing an accident; others can be very serious and long-lasting, such as certain cancers. Most of us learn to accept occasional episodes of nausea and vomiting without undue anxiety, but the symptom itself can be dangerous to certain groups of people, notably diabetics.

If the vomit is black or bloody or you have severe and constant abdominal pain, call a doctor without delay. If significant vomiting follows within forty-eight hours of a head injury, go to your local hospital emergency room.

8.9   Drugs for nausea and vomiting

Three types of drugs can be used. Anticholinergic drugs (8.6(a)) and antihistamines (6.4(a)) affect the vomiting center of the brain. Many are available over the counter; ask the pharmacist about the ingredients in any product you are considering. Low doses of antipsychotic drugs such as Compazine, Stelazine and Thorazine (section 4.12) may be prescribed, usually when vomiting is caused by other drugs or toxic reactions within the body. They have many adverse effects. Antipsychotic drugs in low doses may also be prescribed. Marijuana (cannabis, grass) would be used more to prevent vomiting due to toxic reactions, especially to cancer therapy, if it were legally available (see chapter 3).

8.10   ALTERNATIVES TO DRUGS FOR NAUSEA AND
           VOMITING

If vomiting is associated with diarrhea the cause could be a gut
infection (see section 8.11). Diabetics may require frequent sweetened drinks to keep blood sugar in balance; lemonade is particularly
good, but avoid brands that include synthetic additives. If vomiting
continues, the diabetic will have to be admitted to hospital; this is a
potentially dangerous situation, especially for insulin-dependent diabetics.

Deep, slow breathing and complete relaxation (see section 16.12)
can reduce nausea whatever its cause. If nausea and vomiting are due
to toxic processes within the body—such as cancer and treatments
for it—there are no simple solutions. The best nondrug measures are
those that will tend to improve your general health and enhance your
body's capacity to heal itself.

(a) Travel or motion sickness

Motion sickness can usually be avoided by a combination of strategies. If you are in a car, do not read or look down at anything within
the vehicle for more than a few seconds. Look out the front window.
Fix your head on a suitable headrest and try not to move it. At sea, go
up on deck, breathe deeply and watch the horizon.

Have a light meal shortly before the journey, and eat a little at
frequent intervals during the journey. Ginger can reduce travel sickness, so try chewing ginger candy or eating gingersnaps. Eating carob
candy (from whole-food and health-food stores) may also be helpful.

Parents' attitudes are important in determining whether or not
their children get sick; some children vomit in their parents' car but
not in other people's. Try to think about something other than travel
sickness, and distract children by playing word games, telling stories
or singing. Avoid anxiety about travel sickness; it will make the
problem worse. Teach your children not to worry about it by explain-
ing how to prevent it, and by coping efficiently and promptly whenever it occurs.

(b) Food allergy

Vomiting is sometimes a symptom of food allergy. If it occurs regularly within an hour of eating certain food, the link may be quite easy to detect. Other common symptoms include diarrhea, constipation and abdominal bloating; asthma, hay fever and eczema may develop within a few days to confirm the diagnosis of allergy. Food allergy is more common among children than among adults, and particularly common among those who come from families with other allergic members.

You should be aware that many symptoms of food allergy mimic those of emotional stress, while emotional problems can themselves be both symptoms and promoters of allergy. It can be very difficult to separate the two. See section 18.8 for advice on dealing with food allergy.

8.11   DIARRHEA

Diarrhea is usually self-limiting and of little consequence; it is one of the body's ways of getting rid of unwanted substances as quickly and efficiently as possible. Treatment of acute diarrhea, other than by drinking plenty of liquids (see section 8.13), may actually be harmful if it slows down elimination of toxins or pathogens.

Chronic watery diarrhea can be a symptom of more serious disease. If you have changed your eating habits and your bowels have responded by producing three or more soft motions a day you should not be worried; it is just a new habit to which you will soon become accustomed.

8.12   DRUGS FOR DIARRHEA

Diarrhea treatments usually contain absorbing agents such as kaolin or bulking agents such as methylcellulose. Some also contain drugs which reduce muscular activity in the bowel, such as diphenoxylate; these may make matters worse if the diarrhea is due to infection, because they interfere with the body's efforts to eliminate unwanted organisms. Some doctors may prescribe antibiotics, but this is entirely inappropriate unless you have had a stool test which proves that the diarrhea is caused by bacteria which are sensitive to the antibiotic. When diarrhea is caused by virus infection, antibiotics are worse than useless because they disrupt bowel flora and can cause longer-lasting problems.

Bulking agents (see section 8.15) may be prescribed for chronic diarrhea. Taking these products is equivalent to eating more fiber in your diet, except that high-fiber food also contains other valuable nutrients. It makes sense to eat more high-fiber foods such as whole grains, peas, beans, fruits and vegetables rather than to rely on bulking agents.

8.13   ALTERNATIVES TO DRUGS FOR DIARRHEA

An attack of diarrhea in an adult may be unpleasant but it is usually not a serious matter. You can help your body to cope by drinking more water than usual. If the diarrhea is accompanied by nausea and/or vomiting, eat nothing whatever for twenty-four hours, but drink any fluids you fancy apart from milk, alcohol and coffee.

Diarrhea and vomiting in children are more serious because they can quickly lead to dehydration and loss of essential salts. Children should be encouraged to drink small quantities of liquid very frequently; give them fresh-squeezed orange or lemon juice diluted with water and sweetened with honey, thin soups, jellies and savory vegetable juices, and unlimited pure water. Return gradually to a normal diet when the symptoms have abated.

Recurrent bouts of diarrhea lasting perhaps a day or so are usually caused by anxiety, but they can also be due to inadequate dietary fiber. See section 18.3 for advice.

8.14   CONSTIPATION

One person's normal function is another's constipation. It is very much a matter of what we are used to and what we expect. How often we want to use the toilet varies according to our everyday diet; those who eat large quantities of bulky foods will tend to produce large, soft stools at least once a day, whereas people who choose a highly refined diet or live on processed food may want to go far less often and pass small, hard stools. People in this latter group are likely to complain of constipation and may use laxatives to achieve more frequent motions.

A hundred years ago constipation was believed to be a fearful evil. Our grandparents imagined that it poisoned them from the inside, and that purgatives were essential to counter this horror. Today we know that this is nonsense, though the sort of diet that leads to chronic constipation is hazardous to health because the large intestine can eventually become damaged.

Constipation is likely to be medically important only if it develops in the absence of any change in diet, stress level or life-style. You should consult your doctor (*a*) if you are accustomed to a regular and predictable bowel habit and you start to suffer inexplicable constipation for more than a couple of weeks; (*b*) if you produce very thin, pencillike stools; (*c*) if you suffer abdominal pain and bloating; or (*d*) if you are losing weight unintentionally.

8.15 Drugs for constipation

Five types of drugs are used to treat constipation. Some products contain two different laxative drugs and these appear in two of the lists below.

Stimulant laxatives stimulate the bowel muscle and can cause abdominal cramps. Brand names include Agoral (flavored), Carter's Little Pills, Correctol Tablets, Dialose Plus, Dulcolax, Emulsoil, Evac-U-Gen, Ex-Lax, Feen-a-Mint, Gentle Nature Natural Vegetable Laxative, Modane, Nature's Remedy, Neoloid, Perdiem Granules, Phillips' LaxCaps, Purge Concentrate and Yellowlax.

Saline laxatives are salts of magnesium, sodium or potassium in various mixtures. They cause the bowel contents to retain water, producing a larger stool that is more readily evacuated. Brands include Haley's M-O, Milk of Magnesia and Swan Citroma.

Lubricant laxatives contain mineral oils which soften and lubricate the stools. Brand names include Agoral (plain), Haley's M-O and Milkinol. They are similar in their action to *fecal softeners* such as Colace, Correctol, Dialose, Extra Gentle Ex-Lax, Feen-a-Mint, Geriplex-FS, Kasof, Phillips' LaxCaps, Regutol and Surfac.

Bulking agents increase the bulk of the bowel contents, thereby stimulating the bowel muscles to become active. Many occur naturally in seeds, bran and other vegetable products but there are also semisynthetic forms such as methylcellulose. The following laxatives contain bulking agents: Citrucel, Correctol Natural Grain, Effersyllium, Fiberall, Fibercon, Hydrocil, Maltsupex, Metamucil, Mordane Versabran, Perdiem Granules, Serutan and Syllact.

Regular use of laxatives can lead to addiction. After a while, your bowel will not function without them and it will be difficult to regain a normal bowel habit. In addition, many laxatives disturb the water or mineral balance of the body, while some interfere with the absorption of nutrients from food. All in all, they are best avoided.

8.16 ALTERNATIVES TO DRUGS FOR CONSTIPATION

Long-term constipation is almost always due to inadequate fiber in the diet (see sections 18.2 and 18.3). Drinking too little can also cause it, especially if you are not eating quite as many fruits and vegetables as you should. Try increasing the quantity of water you drink; start the day with a pint of water (as herb tea if you like it), and make sure you take water—not alcohol, coffee or cola—when you are thirsty.

(a) Activity

Constipation can become a real problem if you are inactive or bedridden, and you will have to eat more high-fiber foods to compensate. For those who are mobile, walking stimulates the bowel muscles to function. Running can produce a surprisingly violent need to use the toilet, while bouncing for a few minutes on a minitrampoline will quickly resolve any doubts you might have been feeling about whether you need to go! (See sections 17.2, 17.3 and 17.6.)

(b) Bowel habits

Some people train their bowels to malfunction by ignoring the signals they get from them until the urge that should lead to emptying the bowel all but fades away. If you habitually rush out of the house in the morning without pausing to use the toilet, and are unable to do so for some hours, you have trained yourself to become constipated.

Improved diet and drinking habits will help to remedy this situation, but it may also require some retraining. You need to tune in to the signals from your bowel. Always give yourself plenty of time to use the toilet, and don't expect an immediate evacuation. Try to train yourself to go every morning, after a long drink; and sit on the toilet for half an hour if need be, not straining but waiting quietly for the bowel movement (reading is a sensible habit!). If it does not come even when you give yourself time, try doing stretching, bending and jumping exercises beforehand to stimulate bowel activity. The Royal Canadian Air Force workout (see section 17.6) is ideal.

8.17 SPASTIC COLON OR IRRITABLE BOWEL SYNDROME

This common condition is usually associated with constipation, though some people complain of diarrhea. The symptoms typically vary from time to time; pain may be the worst problem on one occasion, constipation or diarrhea on another. The primary cause is emotional stress, which disrupts the smooth coordination of the contractions of the bowel muscle. It tends to be a recurring problem.

8.18 DRUGS FOR IRRITABLE BOWEL SYNDROME

Doctors are likely to prescribe two types of product: a bulking agent such as methylcellulose (see section 8.15), and antispasmodic drugs which are usually anticholinergics (section 8.6(a)). A few may suggest regular use of laxatives.

The problem with drug treatment is that it often does little to help the sufferer, and indeed may have no beneficial effect at all. If it does seem to help, the outcome is likely to be indefinite dependence on drugs and gradual loss of bowel function.

8.19 ALTERNATIVES TO DRUGS FOR IRRITABLE BOWEL SYNDROME

(a) Diet

Change gradually to a high-fiber diet so that the bowel has sufficient bulk on which to contract (see sections 18.2 and 18.3).

Food allergy, perhaps associated with yeast infection, may be the cause of the problem. Try eliminating the most common trigger foods (see section 18.8) for a couple of weeks to see if the symptoms resolve, then identify the particular foods that affect you and avoid them. Essential fatty acid deficiency is commonly associated with irritable bowel syndrome. Boost your intake of essential fats by following advice in section 18.4(o).

Yeast (candida) infection is particularly likely if your symptoms began within months of a course of antibiotics (see section 5.7) or steroids (sections 6.4(d), 6.8(c) and 7.6). See section 18.6 for dietary advice.

(b) Stress

For four out of five irritable-bowel sufferers, stress can cause a relapse or worsening of symptoms. Regular exercise will help prevent this effect; also, adopt some of the stress management techniques described in chapter 16.

8.20 INFLAMMATORY BOWEL DISEASE

This group includes Crohn's disease, ulcerative colitis and diverticulitis. These conditions are due to problems with the lining of the large intestine. Crohn's disease and ulcerative colitis cause abdominal pain and bloody diarrhea or constipation. Sufferers feel ill, lack energy and lose their appetites. Steroids are often prescribed; their many serious adverse effects are summarized in section 6.4(*d*).

The problem seems to be caused by long-term poor nutrition, leading to excessively low levels of zinc and many vitamins, notably vitamin C and folate. Studies have shown that sufferers eat more sugar and more refined and processed foods than nonsufferers, habitually substituting chemicals for the nutritious foods they need. A varied organic whole-food diet (see section 18.2) will protect you from inflammatory bowel disease and help sufferers to recover from it.

In diverticulitis, little sacs and pockets in the bowel wall become inflamed. They can get infected and produce abdominal pain, nausea and constipation (sometimes diarrhea). If it is very severe, surgery may be necessary to remove the damaged parts of the bowel. Diverticulitis is one of the many adverse consequences of a refined Western diet; it does not occur in countries such as Africa where people habitually eat a high-bulk diet. It can be totally avoided by eating sensibly, and a high-fiber diet is the best treatment (see sections 18.2 and 18.3).

8.21 HEMORRHOIDS

These are enlargements of parts of the lining of the anus. Sometimes they cause pain and sometimes they bleed, leaving a smear of bright red blood on the stool or on the toilet paper.

8.22 DRUGS FOR HEMORRHOIDS

Suppositories and creams for hemorrhoids contain mixtures of some or all of the following ingredients: soothing applications, local anesthetics, astringents and antiseptics. Some are available over the counter and some also on prescription. Over-the-counter brands include Anusol, Medicone, Proctofoam/non-steroid, Tronolane and

Wyanoids. Most are capable of causing local irritation, especially if used frequently. Some preparations also contain steroids (see section 6.4(d)); examples include Analpram-HC, Anusol-HC, Carmol-HC, Cort-Dome, Cortifoam and Proctofoam-HC. Steroids can cause lasting damage to the skin if used regularly for long periods.

8.23 ALTERNATIVES TO DRUGS FOR HEMORRHOIDS

Straining to pass hard stools is the most frequent cause of hemorrhoids, and it will aggravate any problems you may have. The most important consideration is diet. Hemorrhoids are virtually unknown in countries where a high-fiber diet is normal. Follow the advice given for constipation in section 8.16.

Pregnancy can lead to the development of hemorrhoids. Usually they will disappear again after the birth of the baby and cause no further problems.

When hemorrhoids do develop they can continue to cause discomfort even if your life-style is such that you never become constipated and your stools are always soft. Sometimes flare-ups are associated with standing for long periods or with exhaustion. If you can identify the situations which cause problems for you and avoid them, your general health is likely to benefit. If hemorrhoids cause pain when you are using the toilet, try lubricating the anal passage with a little K-Y jelly beforehand. After you have used the toilet, do not rub with hard toilet paper; wash the anal area carefully with lukewarm water. Pat dry and smear zinc and castor-oil cream around the anus.

9

Heart and Blood-Vessel Disease

This chapter deals with common manifestations of heart and blood-vessel (cardiovascular) disease—hypertension (high blood pressure), angina, atheroma and atherosclerosis—and problems caused by inadequate blood supply to the extremities, including leg pain (intermittent claudication), cramps and restless legs, cold and painful extremities, chilblains and Raynaud's disease. The information in this chapter is also important for those who wish to take action to reduce their risk of heart attack, thrombosis or stroke.

Cardiovascular (literally, heart and blood vessel) disease is the most important cause of death and serious disability in the developed countries. In the United States the death toll remains very high even though increased health consciousness—especially the reduction in cigarette smoking—has led to a decline over the past twenty years. Over 40% of American deaths—a million fatalities per year—are due to cardiovascular disease. Many of these deaths are premature.

The seriousness of these conditions and their great prevalence mean that tremendous medical effort goes into treating them. The results of this effort are poor, yet because these diseases are predictable consequences of our Western life-style they are quite readily avoidable. The answer to them does not lie in medical breakthroughs but in changing the way we live. This chapter explains the actions that you can take to do that.

SECTION INDEX

9.1 *The cardiovascular system*

9.2 *Angina and coronary disease*

9.3 *Drugs for angina*

9.4 *Alternatives to drugs for angina*

9.5 *Atherosclerosis (hardening of the arteries) and atheroma*

9.6 *Hyperlipidemia (high blood cholesterol)*

9.7 *Drugs that reduce blood cholesterol*

9.8 *Alternatives to drugs for hyperlipidemia*

9.9 *High blood pressure (hypertension)*

9.10 *Drugs for high blood pressure*

9.11 *Alternatives to drugs for high blood pressure*

9.12 *Restless legs, leg cramps and leg ulcers (peripheral vascular disease)*

9.13 *Raynaud's disease, cold hands and feet, and chilblains*

9.1 THE CARDIOVASCULAR SYSTEM

The cardiovascular system provides the nutrients which are necessary for the survival of every cell in our bodies. When the blood vessels that carry these life-sustaining nutrients fail, the parts that are most seriously deprived will die. This leads to pain and loss of essential functions.

Pain occurs when you put demands on a part that is not getting enough blood. If the vessels feeding your leg muscles are not as good as they should be, you will experience pain with walking. When you stop walking the pain will disappear again. If pain occurs in your heart when you are doing anything that makes it pump faster— whether being physically active or sitting still and getting anxious, angry or upset—it means that the heart needs a better blood supply to feed its own muscle. Blockages in the vessels that feed the heart cause the pain of angina, and if they are sufficiently severe, heart attack.

However, the cardiovascular system is not just a pump and a bunch of pipes that can get blocked up. It responds to hormones and is ultimately controlled by the nervous system. Blood vessels can be opened or closed down in response to commands from nerves in their muscular walls. This means that attention to the physical aspect of their function is not likely to be enough on its own; you must also take action to enhance health on emotional and spiritual levels too. In our materialistic culture the importance to cardiovascular health of these aspects of humanity tends to get ignored, which is why the epidemic of heart disease remains such a mystery to many. It is not enough simply to eat alfalfa sprouts and jog; indeed, such simple-minded measures may be relatively ineffective in your case. Your attitudes and your feelings also crucially affect the way your cardio-vascular system functions.

Each person is different, and this individuality is especially important in relation to cardiovascular health. In order to judge which steps are particularly relevant to you, you will have to assess yourself and your real needs quite carefully.

Beware of following the assumptions that may already have led you into the danger zone; you could do yourself more harm than good. For example, if you are the type of high-achieving person who pushes himself hard, and you have cardiovascular symptoms after a period of pressure at work, the last thing you should do is take up vigorous exercise in an attempt to get yourself fit. You could be pushing yourself into a potentially fatal state of exhaustion. This is the sort of situation that ends with men having heart attacks while out jogging. You must first learn to relax, give yourself time to rest and recuperate, and only then start exercising.

Similarly, you may believe that your weight problem puts you at risk of heart attack. But to react to that threat with a crash diet could make your cardiovascular problem much more serious, because such diets are stressful and can cause abnormal heartbeat patterns. For you, the flab could be less dangerous than the diet, though if you follow our advice on sensible eating and activity you will lose excess weight steadily and thus decrease your risk in a sensible way.

The concept that must be borne in mind is that of *balance*. Cardiovascular health is the product of a balanced life-style, where activity is balanced by relaxation, work balanced by fun, social activity by time to yourself and sedentary hours by physical exercise. The principle holds even on a molecular level: sodium has to be balanced by potassium, carbon dioxide by oxygen, breakdown by rebuilding.

Excess in almost any direction can put you at risk, the risk growing with the length of time that you have been living in an unbalanced way. Our bodies can withstand a great deal of abuse, but the resilience we have when young wears thin over the years. Stress effects gradually accumulate. In Western cultures these effects are clearly measurable. It used to be believed that blood pressure, for example, rose gradually with increasing age. This increase is now acknowledged to be neither natural nor desirable; it is just one of many signs of long-term stress.

The underlying problem is that our systems do not adapt well to the demands of today's world. The checks and balances that were built into our bodies did not anticipate the pressures under which we live now. We suffer stress every time our experience is significantly different from that for which we were designed. Cardiovascular disease is just the dominant form of the resulting breakdown, which is why we are experiencing this epidemic.

If you have turned to this chapter for a specific reason, chances are that you have cause to worry about your cardiovascular system. Perhaps you are taking tablets for high blood pressure; millions do. Perhaps you have been frightened by the death of a near relative.

Perhaps you have been told your blood cholesterol level is too high, or you are getting chest pain. The information given here will help you. It will also keep your whole family healthier. Take your children and your partner with you along the road to better cardiovascular health. They will all benefit.

Our aim is to describe a way of life that will produce health. For this reason we shall not discuss in detail the signs or symptoms of disease. In many cases, anyway, these are irrelevant; you can suffer a heart attack after no warning at all, or after years of treatment for obvious cardiovascular symptoms. The time to take action for cardiovascular health is now, and the action is suitable for everyone, of every age, even those who are probably not at risk. Any improvement in the health of the cardiovascular system will improve your general health; your heart and your blood vessels reflect the overall state of your body.

9.2 ANGINA AND CORONARY DISEASE

Angina is diagnosed when chest pain is associated with effort or emotional arousal. It occurs when the heart muscle is not getting enough oxygen. This is likely to happen when the demand on the heart is high because it is beating harder and faster than normal. If the discrepancy between the heart's need for oxygen and the amount it gets is too great, large parts of the heart muscle will die. This is a heart attack.

Diseased coronary arteries reduce the amount of blood that can reach the heart, so angina may be the first symptom of this problem. However, there is no consistent relationship between damage to the arteries and the development of symptoms. Your arteries may seem quite healthy yet you can still suffer from angina, or you may have no symptoms at all even when the arteries seem almost completely blocked.

Coronary bypass, an operation in which diseased arteries are replaced by healthy ones, is therefore a controversial procedure. Some experts, especially those who view cardiovascular problems rather as a plumber might look at the central-heating system in your home, have great faith in surgery, while those who hold holistic views believe that coronary bypass is usually unnecessary and best avoided.

9.3   DRUGS FOR ANGINA

Two approaches to treatment are used, sometimes both at once. You may be given beta blockers or calcium antagonists to reduce the load on the heart in the hope of preventing angina attacks, and you may also have medication to cut attacks short when they occur.

(a) Beta blockers

Acebutolol (Sectral); atenolol (Tenormin); labetalol (Normodyne, Trandate); metoprolol (Lopressor); nadolol (Corgard); pindolol (Visken); propranolol (Inderal); timolol (Blocadren).

Beta blockers are also produced in combination with diuretics, for example propranolol/hydrochlorothiazide tablets (see section 9.10(b)). Brand names include Inderide, Lopressor HCT, Normozide, Tenoretic and Timolide.

Beta blockers reduce the effect of nervous-system input which would stimulate the heart. Their side effects include excessive slowing of the heart—which can lead to heart failure—cold hands and feet, asthma, leg pain, diabetes, sleep disturbance, nightmares, depression, tiredness, weakness, dry eyes, headache, skin rashes, stomach pain, nausea and vomiting.

If you have been taking beta blockers for more than a week or two it is very important that you do not try to stop them suddenly. A dangerous "rebound" effect can develop, with worsening cardiovascular symptoms and increased risk of heart attack. However, provided that you are *well rested,* and have established yourself on a regime of activity and diet designed to reduce the severity of your cardiovascular problems (see section 9.4), you will be able to cut your intake of beta blockers gradually and get off them safely.

(b) Calcium antagonists

Verapamil (Calan, Isoptin).

These drugs also alter the effects of input to the heart from the nervous system. Side effects include nausea, vomiting, constipation and excessively slow heart rate. They are relatively new drugs and the full range of their effects on the body is not yet known.

(c) Drugs that dilate the blood vessels feeding the heart

Diltiazem (Cardizem); isosorbide dinitrate (Dilatrate, Iso-Bid, Isordil, Isotrate Timecelles, Sorbitrate); nitroglycerin (Deponit NTG Film, Nitro-Bid, Nitrocine, Nitrodisc, Nitro-Dur, Nitrogard Buccal Tablets, Nitroglyn, Nitrol IV, Nitrolingual Spray, Nitrong, Nitrospan, Nitrostat, Transderm-Nitro, Tridil); pentaerythritol tetranitrate (Duotrate, Peritrate, P.E.T.N.).

These drugs allow more blood to reach the heart, thus preventing or cutting short angina attacks. They are relatively safe when used occasionally. Unwanted effects include flushing, headache, dizziness and faintness. Longer-acting preparations can cause swollen ankles.

9.4 ALTERNATIVES TO DRUGS FOR ANGINA

To become free from the pain of angina you need to improve your physical condition so that delivery of oxygen to the heart is more efficient. Stress reduction is also important, both because stress makes you far more vulnerable to angina and because it markedly increases the risk that angina could progress into a full-blown heart attack. Getting rid of the pain with drugs does not prevent you from being at risk. To cure the problem you have to adopt nondrug approaches, restructuring your life to eliminate the causes of your condition.

The first step is to get to know yourself. Learn when your angina occurs and try to avoid it. Keep a diary to help you identify the circumstances under which the pain occurs. Then you will know where to focus your action to increase your resilience.

Each angina attack weakens the heart muscle. To avoid further damage you need to prevent the attacks before they occur. Never push yourself so hard that angina is inevitable, and don't take tablets that will stop the pain so you can go ahead and do something that you know will set it off. Learn to manage without drugs as much as possible.

(a) Rest and relaxation

In many cases the most important immediate cause of angina is the tendency of the coronary arteries to go into spasm, thus cutting off the oxygen supply to the heart. This is a reaction to emotional stress. If your angina occurs frequently you are probably already aware of links between the pain and tiredness or emotional stress. When you are upset or exhausted you may be unable to climb a flight of stairs without angina; when you are well rested you probably don't suffer at all. Angina is often a warning that you need more time off or more sleep, and that you should learn an effective method of relaxation. (See chapter 16 for advice on stress-management techniques.)

(b) Activity

Activity plays a vital part in building your recovery from angina. You have probably become gradually less active because the pain develops with exertion; however, this will tend to make your heart increasingly vulnerable. You should adopt a strategy of slow but steady increments in activity, stopping just short of the point where you expect your angina to start. Obviously, you should not do this until you are well rested. The first step is rest; activity can follow when you have slept as long as you need to sleep and you are feeling relaxed. (See sections 17.1, 17.2, 17.3 and 17.5.)

Avoid all activities that put a sudden strain on the body, such as lifting heavy weights, skiing and similarly demanding types of exercise. Gentle, long-lasting activity is what you need; you can build up speed as your body adapts.

(c) Breathing

Many angina patients breathe in a way that makes their problem more severe. They take too many shallow breaths which do not allow a complete exchange of gases in the lungs, making the circulating blood less rich in oxygen than it should be. This kind of breathing can actually precipitate the spasm in the arteries that causes angina.

Fast breathing is a common response to anxiety. If you tend to feel short of breath this could be at the root of your problem. Fast breathing slides into hyperventilation, often associated with panic attacks, which upsets the chemical balance of the blood, setting off a racing and irregular heartbeat ("palpitations") and putting additional strain on the heart. Whenever an angina attack begins, concentrate on breathing slowly and deeply. This could be enough to cut it short without the need for medication. (See section 16.12 for more details and advice.)

(d) Smoking

Smoking will inevitably make angina worse. It reduces the oxygen content of the blood so that the whole body, including the heart, tends to be deprived of oxygen. In addition it causes the release of the stress hormone epinephrine which speeds up the heart rate and increases the oxygen demand of the heart muscle, making you more vulnerable to angina.

There's no way around this. You have to give it up. If you don't quit you are risking a heart attack. There are many books advising on giving up smoking, but the most important step is to decide that you really are determined to quit. Ask your doctor about local antismoking clinics if you can't break the addiction yourself.

(e) Diet

You have probably been led to believe that your angina is due to deposits of cholesterol in your coronary arteries, and you may have been told to reduce your cholesterol intake. See section 9.8 for advice.

Spasms in the arteries are more probable if your body is short of magnesium. Magnesium is often lacking in our diet because the chemical fertilizers used by conventional farmers prevent plants from taking up sufficient magnesium from the soil. In some places, especially high-rainfall areas with acid soils, the soil can be deficient in magnesium. Acid rain is adding to this problem. You might not be getting quite enough magnesium even from what seems to be an ideal organic whole-food diet. Try a course of supplements of chelated magnesium (from your local health-food store) and incorporate foods rich in magnesium into your everyday diet. See section 18.4(l).

9.5 ATHEROSCLEROSIS (HARDENING OF THE ARTERIES) AND ATHEROMA

Years of inappropriate diet and insufficient activity cause gradual deterioration in the walls of the arteries that deliver blood to every part of the body. Fatty deposits (atheroma) adhere to the arterial walls, forming "plaques" under which ulcers may form. In addition, the vessel walls lose their elasticity, becoming narrowed (stenosed) and rigid. While angina may result from the development of plaques in the coronary arteries, atheroma in other arteries causes damage and pain in other parts of the body. The problem is basically the same whichever artery we consider.

Perhaps the most dangerous aspect of this slow deterioration of the arteries is the fact that it happens silently, without our knowledge. Sudden disaster can strike when a fragile vessel breaks or a clot forms in a damaged artery. The result may be a hemorrhage—bleeding into the tissues—and the parts that were fed by the artery involved will be deprived of essential oxygen and nutrients so they will die. This can happen all over the body, but particular sites are especially vulnerable: in the retina of the eye, tiny arteries can break and bleed, leading to loss of visual acuity and eventually to blindness if the problem is severe; in the brain this process causes strokes, as areas of brain tissue die when their blood supply fails; in the kidney it can lead to loss of function; and in the legs it leads to muscle pain and problems with healing, so you might develop leg ulcers or even gangrene in the toes. All these problems are more severe in heavy smokers and in diabetics, who are especially prone to blood-vessel disease.

Atherosclerosis is most dangerous if it is accompanied by high blood pressure, because pressure on the walls of damaged vessels is particularly likely to lead to rupture. But the two occur together, for pressure needs to rise to force blood through blood vessels narrowed by atherosclerosis. This is a situation that you can avoid by adopting a life-style that will minimize cardiovascular risk *before* you start to suffer symptoms.

The advice given for angina (section 9.4) applies equally to other forms of blood-vessel disease. If you are not actually suffering symptoms, you may be able to take more exercise, and this is very important in the fight against atherosclerosis. Ideally we should all, like our ancestors, walk many miles each day; those who do so are much less likely to suffer any cardiovascular symptoms. (See sections 17.2 and 17.5.)

Follow the dietary advice given in sections 18.2, 18.4(k) and 18.4(n). It is also essential that you give up smoking if you have not already done so. Your problem has primarily to do with lack of oxygen, and smokers' blood contains about 20% less than non-smokers'. In addition, smoking increases the probability of spasm in the arteries.

9.6   HYPERLIPIDEMIA (HIGH BLOOD CHOLESTEROL)

High blood cholesterol is associated with most forms of cardiovascular disease, and is an important factor in the risk of heart attack. People in Western countries have much higher levels of cholesterol in their blood than those in less developed countries. Some individuals have an inherited tendency to develop high levels of cholesterol in the blood; these people are particularly vulnerable to heart disease.

9.7   DRUGS THAT REDUCE BLOOD CHOLESTEROL

These include cholestyramine (Questran), clofibrate (Atromid-S), colestipol (Colestid) and probucol (Lorelco).

The main adverse effects of clofibrate are gallbladder disease, nausea, abdominal pain, itching and impotence. This drug seems to accelerate aging and consequently increases the risk of death from a wide range of causes.

Cholestyramine and colestipol act on the gut, increasing excretion of cholesterol. Side effects include nausea, constipation or diarrhea, heartburn, flatulence, rashes and reduced absorption of vitamins.

9.8 ALTERNATIVES TO DRUGS FOR HYPERLIPIDEMIA

Thanks mainly to the public-relations expertise of the margarine industry, most people believe that high blood cholesterol is caused by eating foods that are high in cholesterol—butter, cheese, eggs and organ meats such as liver. But this is only a small part of the problem; changing to sunflower margarine is therefore not likely to have any marked effect on your blood cholesterol. Recent research shows that fish oils improve the balance of fats in the blood and prevent heart disease. Substitute fish for meat three days a week or take fish oil supplements.

Blood cholesterol rises when stress-hormone levels rise in the body. Like other aspects of cardiovascular disease, the deposition of cholesterol in the arteries is more closely linked with emotional stress than with diet. (See chapter 16 for advice on stress management.) Nevertheless, dietary changes will help, and they will also help you to lose weight, which will reduce the strain on your heart (see sections 18.1, 18.2 and 18.3).

9.9 HIGH BLOOD PRESSURE (HYPERTENSION)

Blood pressure is programed to rise whenever we experience fear, excitement, anger or any other emotional reaction that in our ancestors might have been associated with a need for rapid or forceful movement. Blood pressure is never constant for long, rising and falling with our moods and the demands made upon us. Hypertension, or chronically raised blood pressure, develops when we are exposed too often, or for too long, to the conditions that produce a rise in blood pressure. This is especially true if we are exposed to mental stress without the opportunity for muscular effort. Hypertension is taken seriously by the medical profession because it is associated with an increased risk of heart attack, stroke and other potentially fatal forms of cardiovascular disease. It is not a disease in itself but a symptom that warns of potential hazard.

Blood pressure is tested by measuring the maximum and minimum pressure of blood as it is pumped through the system by the heart. With each beat of the heart there is a surge of blood through the arteries around the body; the pressure of this surge is called systolic pressure. After the surge there is a quiet spell, when the resting pressure in the system can be measured; this is the diastolic pressure. The lower the two measurements are, the longer you can expect to live. If your blood-pressure measurements are consistently over about 140/90 (doctors disagree about the precise cutoff point) you may be diagnosed as hypertensive. With blood pressure over 160/95 you are likely to be prescribed some form of antihypertensive medication.

9.10   DRUGS FOR HIGH BLOOD PRESSURE

A wide range of drugs is used to reduce blood pressure; some are also prescribed for other symptoms of cardiovascular problems.

(a) Beta blockers

Brand names and adverse effects are given in section 9.3(a). These drugs have recently become very popular and are increasingly taking the place of other types of antihypertensives. If you are taking any drug with a name ending in "ol"—such as propranolol—it is probably a beta blocker.

These drugs block the effects on the heart of the stimulating hormone epinephrine. This means that you do not react to stress in the normal way, and your blood pressure will tend to stay low when you are exposed to stress. Do *not* stop taking beta blockers without heeding the warnings in section 9.3(a); you must first reduce your vulnerability to heart attack by following the advice in this chapter.

(b) Diuretics

Diuretics work by causing increased urination, thus reducing blood volume and blood pressure. They may be prescribed at the same time

as beta blockers, sometimes in a combined preparation (marked *
below).

Amiloride hydrochloride (Midamor, Moduretic); bendroflumethiazide (Corzide, Naturetin, Rauzide); bumetanide (Bumex);
chlorothiazide (Aldoclor, Diupres, Diuril); chlorthalidone (Combipres, Demi-Regroton, Hygroton, Tenoretic*, Thalidone); ethacrynic acid (Edecrin); furosemide (Lasix); hydrochlorothiazide
(Aldactazide, Aldoril, Apresazide, Apresoline-Esidrix, Capozide,
Dyazide, Esidrix, Esimil, H-H-R, Hydra-zide, HydroDIURIL, Hydropres, Inderide*, Lopressor HCT*, Maxzide, Moduretic, Normozide*, Oretic, Oreticil, Ser-Ap-Es, Serpasil-Esidrex, Timolide*,
Trandate HCT*, Vaseretic); hydroflumethiazide (Diucardin, Saluron, Salutensin); indapamide (Lozol); methyclothiazide (Aquatensen); metolazole (Diulo, Zaroxolyn); polythiazide (Minizide,
Renese); spironolactone (Aldactazide, Aldactone); triamterene
(Dyazide, Dyrenium, Maxzide).

Diuretics can reduce blood volume excessively, leading to dangerously low blood pressure. They can precipitate the development of
diabetes and make established diabetes worse. Other side effects
include gout, nausea, dizziness, weakness, numbness, pins and needles, skin rashes, blood disorders, liver damage, allergic reactions and
impotence. Most diuretics cause increased excretion of potassium,
leading to disturbance of heartbeat, increased toxicity of drugs,
muscle weakness, constipation and loss of appetite. Potassium supplements may be given with certain diuretics. These can cause nausea, vomiting and ulcers. Certain diuretics (notably spironolactone
and triamterene) cause potassium to be conserved in the body;
potassium supplements must *never* be taken with these.

(c) Other antihypertensive drugs

The drugs described below are most often used when beta blockers
and diuretics are insufficient to keep blood pressure down. They may
be given as part of a cocktail of three or four different types of drug,
but this can be a dangerous strategy because the risk of adverse
reactions rises with the number of drugs taken. Some of the products
in the lists below contain more than one type of drug; for example,
Minizide contains both a diuretic and a vasodilator. If you are in

doubt about what your tablets contain, ask your pharmacist or consult a book such as the *Physicians' Desk Reference* (PDR).

1. *Vasodilators*: diazoxide (Proglycem), hydralazine, minoxidil (Loniten), prazosin (Minipress, Minizide), sodium nitroprusside (Nipride, Nitropress).

   These drugs reduce blood pressure by dilating the blood vessels. Adverse effects include fluid retention, weight gain, nausea and vomiting. Existing angina may be aggravated.

2. *Centrally acting antihypertensives*: methyldopa (Aldoclor, Aldomet, Aldoril) has over a hundred known adverse effects, affecting all body systems. Serious hazards are blood disorders and liver damage. Other side effects include impotence, sedation, weakness, depression, nightmares, nausea, dry mouth, stuffy nose, stomach upsets, diarrhea, constipation, fever, dizziness, skin rashes and joint pain. It can also aggravate angina.

   Clonidine hydrochloride (Catapres, Combipres) reduces arousal, and may thus cause drowsiness. Other hazards include dizziness, depression, headache, insomnia, nausea, euphoria, fluid retention, slow heartbeat and chilblainlike spasms of arteries feeding hands and feet. Sudden discontinuation of long-term therapy can cause agitation and a dangerous rise in blood pressure.

   Reserpine and related drugs (Demi-Regroton, Diupres, Hydromox, Hydropres, Metatensin, Naquival, Raudixin, Rauwiloid, Rauzide, Regroton, Renese, Salutensin, Ser-Ap-Es, Serpasil) can cause deep depression and is believed to have been responsible for suicides. Other adverse effects are similar to those of clonidine (above). Some of these products contain a diuretic (9.10(*b*)) as well as reserpine; they may cause adverse effects of both types of drug.

3. *Guanethidine* (Esimil, Ismelin); *phenoxybenzamine hydrochloride* (Dibenyline). Adverse effects of these drugs can include dizziness and fainting on rising (postural hypotension), failure of ejaculation, nasal congestion and gastrointestinal problems.

4. *Captopril* (Capoten, Capozide) reduces resistance to blood

flow in small vessels, thus reducing blood pressure. It can damage the bone marrow, increasing vulnerability to serious infection. If you are taking this drug and you notice any symptoms of infection (e.g., sore throat), *consult your doctor without delay*. Other adverse reactions include skin disease and kidney damage; also loss of taste, mouth inflammation, abdominal pain and dizziness.

5. *Enalapril* (Vaseretic, Vasotec) works in much the same way as captopril (above); it is said to produce fewer serious adverse effects but it is a relatively new drug and its problems may not yet be known.

9.11   ALTERNATIVES TO DRUGS FOR HIGH BLOOD PRESSURE

The basic problem with all antihypertensive drugs is that the body will try to reduce their effects by raising the blood pressure. Taking drugs for this condition is rather like adjusting the thermometer when the temperature is too high; they suppress the symptom but leave the cause untouched. Inevitably, blood-pressure control will be less effective as time goes on, while the risk of adverse effects will rise steadily. But very high blood pressure must be reduced to avoid damage to small, delicate blood vessels, particularly those in the eyes and kidneys. Do not give up taking your drugs until you have adopted the life-style changes that will remove the cause of this symptom.

Those cardiologists who believe that drug therapy for high blood pressure is generally unwise find that they are almost always able to teach their patients to reduce their own blood pressure without medication. The wisdom of their approach is clear both from the accumulating evidence of the widespread problems of adverse effects of antihypertensive drugs and from studies that have shown little or no long-term benefit from drug treatment in all but the most severely hypertensive patients. Indefinite drug therapy is rarely the wisest course of action. Many other approaches are possible, but you will need to use them in concert to achieve a long-term reduction in blood pressure.

(a) Relaxation

Stress is the most common and most important reason for high blood pressure. Your problem may be overwork, insufficient sleep, inability to relax or unhappiness at work or at home. If you stand back and consider your life you are probably able to identify the major cause of your stress.

You will have to take time for yourself to deal with this problem. You may have some serious decision-making to do; if you don't protect yourself better, the consequences could be dire. Ask yourself these questions: Are you in the right job? Are you expecting too much of yourself? Can you work a shorter week, delegate more responsibility to others, take on fewer commitments, resign from committees, make yourself less available to others? A counselor may be able to help you clarify the issues that are threatening your health and to work out the priorities in restructuring your life.

Meditation, yoga and relaxation exercises are all capable of reducing blood pressure. Read all of chapter 16 and adopt a stress-reducing regime that suits you.

(b) Salt (sodium)

High blood pressure has been convincingly linked with the high-salt diet that is characteristic of developed countries, and salt restriction is often recommended as part of the strategy for reducing blood pressure. The average salt (sodium) intake in the West vastly exceeds physiological requirements, while there is a relative lack of potassium in our diet (see section 18.4(n)).

If your blood pressure problem is severe, if you are elderly or black, salt restriction alone could produce a significant drop in blood pressure. There is a wide variation in individual response to sodium salt in the diet; it affects some people more than others, and some races more than others. If your hypertension is only slight, there may be no apparent effect, but a reduction in salt will benefit your health anyway. If you are taking antihypertensive drugs, reducing your salt intake is likely to mean you can reduce the dosage of the drugs.

Unsalted food seems tasteless to many people, especially those under stress; we have become accustomed to a highly salted diet. Guides to the sodium content of common foods are available from pharmacists and bookstores, but see section 18.12 for more advice. Many preparations for indigestion are very high in sodium. Try to avoid using them (see sections 8.3 and 8.4). Relaxation—especially around mealtimes—will help to prevent indigestion, as will adopting a healthier diet.

(c) Excess weight

Blood pressure rises with increasing body weight. Some hypertensives can overcome their problem just by losing weight. However, for many this proves very difficult; they lose some weight on a slimming diet but then find that it goes right on again afterward, and the diet seesaw becomes a depressing and pointless business. They find that fat increases apparently inexorably, while stress levels rise with the struggle.

Alcohol and, unfortunately, many antihypertensive drugs will make your weight problem worse. Give up drinking alcohol if you can; if your work involves alcohol at lunches, change to low sodium mineral waters. Often the desire for alcohol is related to stress; again, the answer could lie in adopting antistress measures.

Weight loss is important if you have rolls of excess fat around your waist, or a large belly, but you are not likely to lose it by depriving yourself of the nutritious food you need. Instead, follow the strategy described in section 10.8.

(d) Activity

Studies of people who take up regular physical activity reveal that it is an effective means of reducing blood pressure. Fairly strenuous exercise such as swimming and jogging will push your blood pressure up while you are active, but when you relax afterward your blood pressure will fall and it will stay down for at least twenty-four hours. Choose types of activity that you can do for at least half an hour at a time, preferably every day. Always take care with exercise; you should not push yourself too hard. Don't increase the demands on your body if you are exhausted. Don't squeeze a heavy session in the gym into an already overcrowded day. You must first build more time for yourself into each day; you need time for both activity and relaxation. (See chapter 17 for advice.)

(e) Dealing with destructive emotions

The most potent generators of chronic high blood pressure are destructive emotional states—particularly anger, resentment and frustration. These emotions produce dangerous stress hormones.

Are you struggling in a job where your efforts are not appreciated? Perhaps you need to sacrifice part of your income in order to achieve greater job satisfaction. Can you move into a different part of the organization, or into a less stressful post elsewhere? Do you need to take your work, or that difficult supervisor (who is probably hypertensive too!), so seriously? Are you setting inappropriately high standards for yourself, or expecting yourself to achieve ambitions that may not be right for you? Have you set yourself an unrealistic timetable? Hypertension is a warning that some sort of shift—in attitudes at least—is essential to your health.

Marital disharmony may be at the root of your problem. A moribund or unsatisfying relationship is a time bomb ticking away under your health. If this is your situation, you must take action. Build up your emotional reserves with antistress measures and increased physical activity, and seek a counselor.

You may have to face a short-term crisis before you can achieve better long-term prospects. Make sure that you are able to weather the crisis by taking sufficient time for yourself and by building up your physical resilience. Don't try to do everything at once when your body is already showing signs of strain.

(f) Pets

Simply stroking a pet reduces blood pressure. A cat will soothe you with its purring, and a dog will make you feel wanted even when the world rejects you. Pets may be troublesome on occasion, but pet owners know that the rewards more than compensate. Is it time you added an animal to your household?

(g) Attitudes

When we get trapped by destructive emotions or a stressful way of life what we often most need is to find a new way of seeing ourselves and our situation. Focus on things that give you hope—they may be the plants growing in your greenhouse or a total life philosophy—and try to regenerate your love of life and of yourself. Have the strength to forget those things that seem to trap you, the oughts, the duties; turn your back on them and walk away. You have nothing to save but your life.

9.12   RESTLESS LEGS, LEG CRAMPS AND LEG ULCERS (PERIPHERAL VASCULAR DISEASE)

These problems are associated with poor circulation to the leg muscles. When muscles get a poor supply of oxygen and nutrients, they cease to function normally and become susceptible to cramp. Too little blood reaching the skin and feet leads to the death of the cells, resulting in slow healing of wounds on the legs and feet, numb toes, loss of hair growth on the feet and toes, leg ulcers and ultimately gangrene. The answer is the same whatever the precise symptoms. Adopt the preventative strategy described in section 9.4. You will get the bonus of a reduced risk of stroke or heart attack.

(a) Activity

Cramps and restless legs at night can be helped by an evening walk. The more miles you cover, the more your legs will benefit. However, if you are a committed exerciser and you run or do other strenuous activity using the legs on a regular basis, your problem could be related to overuse and exhaustion in the muscles. Try exercising earlier in the day and a little more gently.

Stretching the calf muscles can ease restless legs. Try this exercise. Stand in your bare feet and face a wall about eighteen inches away. Lean toward the wall, holding your body straight and keeping your heels flat on the floor. You will feel the pull in your calves. Hold that position for a count of ten, stand straight and relax for ten seconds, then lean again. As you grow accustomed to this exercise you will be able to repeat it more often.

When you have done your walk and exercises and you are ready for bed, lie on your back on the floor or on a firm bed. Lift your legs from the hips until your feet point to the ceiling. Hold this pose to assist the drainage of blood from your legs. They will feel more relaxed afterward.

Young people and others who have perfectly healthy arterial blood supply can suffer from restless legs. The cause in such cases is often muscular tension, usually resulting from emotional tension or an overactive mind. Ease the tension in the short term by relaxing in a warm bath before you retire; in the longer term, take up running or some other form of regular aerobic exercise which will relax your whole body, and find a stress-releasing method such as meditation that works for you. (See chapter 16.)

(b) Smoking

This is the most common cause of peripheral vascular disease. If you are in any doubt about the link between cigarette smoking and arterial disease, just pay a visit to the men's surgical ward of your local hospital. There you will see bed after bed occupied by heavy smokers whose legs have to be amputated because the blood supply is inadequate. You will probably not find a single lifetime nonsmoker there. In Germany they call arterial damage to the legs "the smoker's disease."

9.13 RAYNAUD'S DISEASE, COLD HANDS AND FEET, AND CHILBLAINS

These unpleasant conditions are related to the sort of blood-vessel problems discussed above, but they can occur in people whose arteries are apparently quite healthy. They are due to problems with the nervous control of the blood vessels; the arteries shut down too far in response to cold or other stimuli and do not readily open up again. Certain drugs can cause these problems. Beta blockers are the most common culprits, but other antihypertensives may be to blame. Cannabis (marijuana) and nicotine may make matters worse.

In Raynaud's disease, sudden attacks of cold and pallor in the extremities—usually fingers and toes—can occur in response to cold, emotion or vibration. This is caused by constriction of the small arteries near the surface of the skin, and it can last from a few minutes to an hour or more.

Strategies that improve cardiovascular health are likely to be helpful. Pay special attention to diet; magnesium is particularly important (see section 18.4(l)), but a generally good micronutrient balance will reduce irritability in the nervous system (see sections 18.2 and 18.4(n)). Exercise will help too. Problems with cold feet in otherwise reasonably healthy people can be cured completely when they take up regular running. Any form of activity that makes the feet markedly warm will improve peripheral circulation and reduce the problem of arterial spasm; running, with its combination of increased cardiac output, muscular enhancement of circulation and repeated contact with the ground, is undoubtedly the most effective (see section 17.7). Less strenuous exercise may make little appreciable difference, although it will tend to slow down deterioration.

Problems with circulation to the hands are best dealt with by adopting the nearest parallel to running—sawing wood or weight training with dumbbells. When we cease to use the muscles of our hands and arms the circulation becomes less efficient and less well controlled. You need to reverse this trend in your own life if you suffer from Raynaud's disease or chilblains.

Clearly it makes sense also to avoid stimuli that precipitate attacks of cold. Cold itself is the most common, so warm woolen socks—particularly at night—insulated insoles in your shoes, even the electrically heated socks worn by motorcyclists, could be the answer for cold feet; if you suffer when your hands get cold you should go to some trouble to ensure that you always have efficient gloves (ski shops offer the best available). And if despite your precautions, you still get cold, then warm hands or feet slowly in tepid water. Hotter water is liable to cause pain.

Vibration from tools or machinery is capable of causing long-term nerve damage, and Raynaud's disease could be the first symptom you experience. If this is the case you must stop using the tools that damage you. There is no alternative. Nerve damage can be progressive and irreversible, so it must be taken seriously.

10

Metabolic Problems

This chapter is concerned with diabetes, hypoglycemia and obesity.

SECTION INDEX

10.1 *Metabolism: what is it and what controls it?*
10.2 *Diabetes*
10.3 *Drugs for diabetes*
10.4 *Alternatives to drugs for diabetes*
10.5 *Hypoglycemia*
10.6 *Obesity*
10.7 *Drugs for obesity*
10.8 *Alternatives to drugs for obesity*

10.1 METABOLISM: WHAT IS IT AND WHAT CONTROLS IT?

Metabolism concerns the basic processes by which molecules of food are broken down and used to release energy and to build tissue. This is something that goes on in every part of us, and it is largely controlled by sophisticated chemical messenger systems which in turn are regulated by the brain's hormone master gland, the pituitary. It is a system in which every part affects every other part; where any change will have many ramifications; and through which anything that happens in our minds can produce effects in the furthest parts of our bodies.

Medicine tends to deal with metabolic processes as if they were relatively constant. Metabolic malfunction, once established, is likely to be looked upon as though it were there forever; a metabolic illness such as diabetes is therefore seen as an immutable problem which must be kept under control by indefinite treatment with drugs. In reality our metabolic processes vary constantly, from day to day and from hour to hour; we respond to changes in demand, to the imposition of stress and to its relaxation. We establish a new balance to fit each new circumstance; there may be some delay as the body adapts, as with jet lag, but such adaptation as is possible for each individual will eventually occur.

Some metabolic problems, however, are beyond the reach of adaptation. When a gland ceases to secrete an essential hormone such as insulin, or when the adrenal cortex ceases to produce its hormones (after years of exposure to steroid drugs, for example), it may be impossible to persuade it to function normally again. If any of these chemical regulators of metabolism ceases to be available to the body, death is the final outcome unless it is replaced. In this area recent advances in medicine have been invaluable; millions of people are kept alive by replacement therapy.

A health-promoting way of living is particularly essential for such people. The replacement hormones are never available in the precise quantities that are needed, nor at the precise time they are needed, and they are never quite as effective as they should be. Balance must be carefully maintained by a way of living that maximizes the efficiency of metabolic function. Those who depend on replacement therapy for survival must look after themselves more carefully than other people.

A wide variety of metabolic problems is actually caused by drug therapy. If you take medicine regularly to change one aspect of your biochemical balance—for example, to reduce the amount of water in your body to cut the load on your heart—your whole body will adapt to this medicine. But sometimes this adaptation causes further problems as you develop a drug-induced metabolic imbalance. Indeed, as one expert pointed out in the *British Medical Journal, all* drug-induced disease is metabolic.

Obviously the way to avoid suffering from metabolic disease caused by drug therapy is to avoid using drugs, or if you need to use them, to manage with the absolute minimum. To counter the effects of drug-induced metabolic imbalance you should eat a good balanced diet (see section 18.2) and boost your intake of foods that aid the liver's detoxifying function (18.5(*a*)). This increases your chances of health in the face of the metabolic disruption that drugs induce.

10.2   DIABETES

The body needs a constant level of sugar in the blood to fuel cells and provide energy. It manufactures sugar for this purpose from the food we eat. When blood sugar falls, new supplies are released from body stores; when it rises after we eat, the pancreas, a large gland near the stomach, produces insulin, which allows cells to take up sugar from the blood for immediate use or for storage. If the pancreas ceases to produce insulin (usually for unknown reasons, though virus infection and immune-system malfunction are probably involved) the body becomes starved of sugar and the most severe form of diabetes results. It is diagnosed when the blood sugar level is abnormally high and unused sugar is discharged in the urine. It is particularly likely to happen during childhood or adolescence, and the condition is often called *juvenile-onset diabetes*. Other names are *insulin-dependent* and *type I diabetes*.

These names distinguish this type of illness from another form which is now common: *adult onset* or *type II diabetes*. This usually develops in adults who are or have been overweight, and it is due to resistance in the cells to insulin. Most of these diabetics produce normal or even high levels of insulin, but it does not have a normal effect.

The two forms of diabetes are different in many ways. Juvenile-onset diabetes can produce rapid wasting as the body burns fat as a substitute for the sugar it cannot use without insulin. This leads to the accumulation of poisons (ketones) in the blood and eventually to coma and death unless insulin is injected. Sufferers feel very weak and thirsty, with aches and pains throughout the body. Often they smell strongly of acetone (as in nail-polish remover). Mature-onset diabetes develops gradually. Many middle-aged or elderly diabetics are unaware of illness, though it may be picked up in health screening. Sometimes it comes to their doctors' attention because of problems with healing or infection; a persistent leg ulcer or boils may be the first sign of metabolic disturbance.

Both types of diabetes are becoming steadily more common. Diabetes among children is now six times more common than it was thirty years ago. It is one of many ways in which our bodies break down under the stresses of modern life.

10.3   DRUGS FOR DIABETES

(a) Insulin

Type I diabetics must have insulin. It is taken by injection since stomach acids destroy it. Many forms of insulin are available and they have different metabolic effects, although all play broadly the same role in the body. The dose has to be worked out carefully for each diabetic and it may vary slightly from day to day as requirements change. If they are to live normal, minimally restricted lives, diabetics must become capable of judging their insulin needs, the timing of their injections and the suitability of particular types of insulin; the precision with which they must judge their internal state requires that they know themselves very well. Devices for testing blood sugar and urine levels are useful aids to the development of this essential self-knowledge. By comparing the test readings with their own internal cues, diabetics can learn to sense the changes in their blood sugar. Important cues include the feelings of lethargy, weakness, irritability and thirst that signal the need for insulin, and the hunger that warns of an excessively low blood sugar level that must be corrected with food.

Insulin is a natural product of the body, but too much of it will kill. Hypoglycemia, or low blood sugar, results when a diabetic has too little carbohydrate to balance the injected insulin. If sugar is not taken quickly, hypoglycemia will cause irritability, disorientation and hallucinations followed by coma. This will progress to brain starvation and death unless glucose is injected.

Some diabetics react adversely to particular insulins; if the insulin they are using does not suit them, their blood sugar control may be poor and they may suffer aches and pains and feel generally under par. Even a change from acid to buffered insulin can cause problems, while a change from ox to pig or human insulin may completely throw off the delicate blood sugar balance. Different insulins vary in a range of important ways.

Human insulin, produced by genetic engineering, is increasingly widely used. Some doctors believe that human insulin should always be used, but some diabetics respond badly to it. Human insulin brands include Humulin, Novolin and Velosulin Human.

Natural insulin is slightly acid; brands include Insulin Injection USP, Iletin and Velosulin. Manufacturers often add substances which reduce the acidity of insulin; this is said to prevent discomfort during injection, although no diabetic we have asked experiences problems with acid insulin. Neutral insulins include NPH Iletin and NPH Purified Pork Insulin.

Many insulins are modified by the addition of zinc and other substances so that they act for longer than the forms above, and fewer injections are required. It is rarely possible to achieve the same precision of blood sugar balance with these insulins. Brand names include Iletin I (Lente, Semilente and Ultralente), Lente Insulin, Protamine, Semilente Insulin, Ultralente Insulin and Zinc & Iletin I.

(b) Tablets

The following drugs are prescribed for type II diabetes: acetohex-amide, chlopropamide (Diabenese), glipizide (Glucotrol), tolazamide (Tolinase), tolbutamide (Orinase). These drugs reduce the level of sugar in the blood but cannot replace insulin. Instead they stimulate the pancreas to produce more insulin. Their adverse effects include weakness, headaches, skin rashes, blood disorders and jaundice. However, the most common problem with tablets for diabetes is hypoglycemia.

A major study in the United States has revealed that diabetics treated with tablets are more likely to die than those prescribed insulin or simply advised to change their diet. If you take these drugs you would be wise to follow the advice on alternatives below so that you can control your diabetes without tablets.

10.4 ALTERNATIVES TO DRUGS FOR DIABETES

Whatever type of diabetic you are, there is much you can do to reduce the seriousness of your illness and avoid some of its long-term complications. Although few type I diabetics will be able to change their metabolism sufficiently to need no treatment at all—there is no alternative to insulin if your body is incapable of producing it—it may be possible to cut insulin requirements; the less insulin you use to keep your blood sugar down to normal levels the better your long-term prospects. Any change in therapy for diabetes must be made very slowly and carefully. All the time you must listen closely to feedback from your body about what you are doing.

If you have been diabetic since childhood you are probably able to adjust your insulin use in response to changing needs. As you alter your life-style, try dropping the quantity by one unit and see how you feel after a couple of days on this lower dose. If your blood sugar stays down, continue reducing medication very slowly. Test your urine or blood sugar regularly during this adjustment process, but *take care;* don't ever try to change too much or too fast.

It is essential to understand that each diabetic is different, and that nobody can tell you exactly how you will react to events in your life, to internal changes and to environmental stimuli. You must know yourself and how you react. This knowledge comes from faith in yourself and cautious experimentation. The greatest hurdle could be the change in attitude that enables you to stop being simply a patient who follows given rules and become a confident person capable of responding appropriately to your own needs.

This self-monitoring strategy will be made easier if you can minimize the fluctuations in your blood sugar level. Reducing your need for insulin is one way of doing this and a reason why it is so important. A regular routine will also help. Getting up at the same time every morning, eating the same breakfast and going through the same general pattern without wide variations will allow your body to function in a consistent way from day to day.

(a) Diet

All diabetics are told to watch their diets, but ideas about the best diet have recently changed dramatically and some diabetics are still following discredited rules which actually increase the severity of their illness. You should eat a high-fiber diet, with large quantities of unrefined carbohydrate foods (see section 18.3). We cannot give rules about precise quantities, nor should you follow anybody's rules but your own, since your body's reactions to what you eat will vary. What is important is that you eat the *types* of food that will give you plenty of natural fiber. Oatmeal (no sugar!), peas and beans are particularly good.

You will also benefit from a diet that contains high levels of chromium (section 18.4(m)), magnesium (18.4(l)), manganese (18.4(k)), zinc (18.4(j)), vitamin C (18.4(f)) and nicotinic acid (18.4(c)). Organic whole foods will keep your micronutrient levels higher (18.2). Supplements of brewer's yeast, which is a particularly rich source of chromium, can be helpful, but you should monitor your blood sugar carefully if you start taking yeast tablets, because they can reduce insulin requirements markedly. While this is beneficial, you may need to adapt your medicine use to take account of the change.

If you are a type II diabetic you will probably be able to give up insulin and tablets within weeks if you change to a diet containing 60% natural carbohydrate foods (see sections 18.2 and 18.3), while type I diabetics can reduce their insulin needs by an average of 25%

and suffer fewer episodes of hypoglycemia. As an added advantage, blood cholesterol levels also fall.

All diabetics should try to avoid sugar and anything that contains processed sugar, such as candy, cookies, cakes, jam and puddings and the most popular sources of sugar. However, if you develop hypo-glycemia (characterized by confusion that often mimicks drunken-ness, a pale yellowish complexion, dark rings around the eyes and a thumping heart) you need sugar *immediately,* and you should have a jar of honey to meet this need when it arises.

When vomiting makes it difficult to hold down sufficient food to balance insulin, sweet drinks—especially lemonade—will help. You may need to go to a hospital emergency room for a glucose injection if hypoglycemia seems unavoidable.

(b) Exercise

The more active you are the less insulin you need and the lower the risk you run of long-term complications of diabetes. So a high level of activity is good for all diabetics. If you take insulin by injection you will have to monitor carefully the effects of a marked boost in activity levels and make sure you eat enough food to compensate for the extra energy you are using. Extended activity such as a day's hiking requires careful planning and plenty of sandwiches and fruit to keep your blood sugar on an even keel. If you take up a strenuous activity such as running, if possible go with a companion who can watch for signs of hypoglycemia and act appropriately.

CAUTION: If you are taking insulin you must not simply stop using it. You need to know to what degree you are dependent on it. If you are in any doubt about the nature of your diabetes ask your specialist for more information and enlist his help in reducing your insulin use.

If you suffer from type II diabetes and you take up a program of regular activity combined with the sort of diet described above, you can expect to become free from symptoms within a matter of weeks, or a year at the most if you are markedly overweight. Consult sections

17.2, 17.3 and 17.4 for advice on suitable types of activity and don't hesitate to follow it; it could add years to your life!

10.5　HYPOGLYCEMIA

Hypoglycemia (low blood sugar) does not affect only diabetics. It is a significant cause of road accidents, learning disabilities and many supposedly "neurotic" symptoms among nondiabetics. Many people will be familiar with the pattern of confusion, faintness, fatigue, headache, blurred vision, palpitations, weepiness, panic and poor circulation that is characteristic of hypoglycemia. Chronic dieters are particularly susceptible, as are those who habitually eat sugary snacks (and who may be on the brink of developing diabetes) and those who miss meals or go to work without an adequate breakfast.

Smoking, alcohol, coffee and certain medicines, notably Flagyl and beta blockers (see section 9.3(a)) are liable to cause hypoglycemia. Try to avoid all of these. If you drink heavily and decide to stop, be especially careful to eat in a way that will protect you from hypoglycemia.

(a) Diet

It is very important that you eat frequently. Have six small meals a day rather than a few large ones, but don't eat more food than you want—just spread it out more evenly. Of course, you should not go hungry either; that's just asking for trouble. If you feel hungry, don't delay or have a cigarette; eat.

Eat more unrefined, complex carbohydrate foods. A high-fiber diet (see section 18.3) is suitable for hypoglycemics because it keeps the blood sugar level steady. Make sure you get enough chromium (section 18.4(m)) and nicotinic acid (18.4(c)). Don't eat sugar at all. Don't use artificial sweeteners; these can cause hypoglycemia by stimulating the pancreas to release insulin even though your body may not need it, because we are conditioned to react to sweet tastes with insulin production and a reduction of blood sugar. If your body reacts very strongly to sugar you will be particularly susceptible to hypoglycemia. You are liable to have problems also with honey, concentrated apple juice, dried fruit and other forms of concentrated natural sugars. The answer for you is to avoid anything that tastes any sweeter than a raw carrot—at least until your body establishes a better balance.

(b) Stress

Stress increases susceptibility to hypoglycemic attacks. If you are going into a situation that you may find stressful, make sure you have a meal first. Remember to eat during long days of shopping or driving, and always take some food with you if you are staying away from home or going anywhere where there may be long gaps between meals.

Guard against the effects of stress by taking plenty of B-group vitamins (see section 18.4(b)). Yeast tablets and yeast spreads are good sources.

10.6 OBESITY

It is regrettably true that one of the most common reasons for persistent weight problems is dieting to lose weight. Dieting makes you fat. To become slim requires a completely different approach.

Obesity has two main dietary causes. The first is malnutrition due to lack of attention to actual food needs—eating foods your body does not need, eating foods that do not provide sufficient nourishment, eating when what you really want is emotional solace, and refusing food when you do need it. The second cause is loading your body with chemicals—drugs, food additives and pesticide residues, refined sugar, household products and industrial chemicals. If you are taking in more than your body can cope with, it can react by storing chemicals and their breakdown products in fat. Inactivity makes it even harder for your body to handle poor diet and a heavy chemical load.

Dieting has many dangers. By constantly overriding the messages from your body about the food you want to eat, you distort your whole relationship with food. It becomes difficult to tune in to what you really need. In addition, dieting reduces your detoxification capacity, making it more difficult to handle the chemicals which are ubiquitous in our environment. Worse than that, when you lose weight by dieting you lose lean tissue; when you put the weight back on (because you can't keep yourself deprived forever) you put on fat. So gradually the proportion of fat in your body rises. At the same time your body's metabolic rate falls, so you eat less and less while growing fatter and fatter.

10.7   DRUGS FOR OBESITY

Drug treatment for obesity has been condemned by many medical experts for years, yet some doctors will still give in to pressure from desperate people. Drugs usually work in the short term, just as most diets do, but in the long term they are not an effective answer.

Three main types of drugs are used to promote weight loss. The first consists of stimulants which suppress the appetite; amphetamine ("speed," no longer available from responsible doctors) is the archetype. Drugs such as diethylpropion (Tenuate, Tepanil), mazindol (Mazanor, Sanorex), phentermin (Adipex-P, Fastin, Ionamin, Oby-Trim, Span R/D, T-Diet, Teramine), while less dangerous than amphetamines, are also addictive stimulants. All drugs of this type are capable of inducing agitation, sleeplessness, gastrointestinal problems, dizziness and psychotic episodes. Over-the-counter appetite suppressants may contain the same stimulant drugs as decongestants (see section 5.5); they are dangerous to people with cardiovascular problems.

The second type of drug is fenfluramine (Pondimin). This is not a stimulant, though it also suppresses appetite. Its adverse effects include drowsiness, dry mouth, dizziness, nausea, fatigue and aching pains. It causes unpredictable emotional changes, disturbed sleep and vivid dreams.

Thirdly there are bulk-forming drugs, usually based on methylcellulose, which claim to help weight reduction by inducing a feeling of satiety. Some of these are available over the counter from pharmacies. However, since appetite has little to do with how full one's belly feels, they are usually ineffective; the body is not fooled so easily.

10.8 ALTERNATIVES TO DRUGS FOR OBESITY

(a) Diet

Reducing the amount of food you eat is ineffective as a long-term strategy, but changing the *type* of food you eat will help you lose excess weight. You should eat enough food to meet your body's needs so that you do not feel hungry or deprived. Don't count calories or avoid high-calorie foods—don't even think about calories. Go for a balanced whole-food diet as described in section 18.2. Make sure you eat plenty of unrefined carbohydrates. Cut down on cheese, use only skim or soya milk and avoid red meat. Eat lots of vegetables, fish, nuts and grains. Avoid all processed foods, all "diet" foods, all foods containing artificial sweeteners, and anything containing the additives listed in section 18.10. Have no refined foods such as those prepared from white flour.

Above all, eat when you are hungry and stop when you are satisfied! When you want to nibble, go ahead and nibble, but ask yourself before you start what you *really* want to eat. Tune into your needs at that particular time, then eat as your body tells you. Beware of false signals like a desire for chocolate or sugar; they mean you need nourishment. Get it from nutritious foods such as nuts, grains, vegetables and free-range or country eggs.

(b) Raising your metabolic rate

If you have been dieting for a long time you may have discovered that you need very little food to maintain your weight. You probably fear that if you ate as often as we suggest, and stopped worrying about calories, you would put on huge amounts of fat very fast. Your weight problem in fact is related to a low metabolic rate and a thrifty metabolism, which means that your body does not burn food as fast as most people's. But you don't need to accept a low metabolic rate. Your body has adjusted to conditions of famine—which is what dieting is as far as your metabolism is concerned. What you must do is persuade your body that food is not short so that your metabolic rate can rise from the depressed level it is at. By changing your lifestyle you can induce changes in your metabolic rate that could allow you to eat three times as much food as you do today—without putting on fat. And you will feel very much better for it.

This is why it is especially important for you to get in touch with your real food needs and to eat in response to hunger, not to deny it. It may take some time for you to accept your needs, but persevere; your body will tell you how much you require to stay healthy—which means reasonably slim.

The most effective way of raising your metabolic rate is by increasing your activity level and eating plenty of protein and micronutrients; nuts and seeds are excellent sources, as are eggs and fresh "oily" fish such as herring. As your metabolic rate rises you are likely to find you do not suffer so much from the cold and you have more energy. You will be able to expend more energy on all your everyday activities and be happy to build more activity into your life. This in turn will raise your metabolic rate higher.

At the beginning of this process it is possible that you will put on some weight. Don't worry about that—don't even think about it. This is a long-term approach, and short-term fluctuations are of no consequence. So don't even bother to weigh yourself; you're not going to act on that information any more; use instead the internal cues that you have probably been trying to ignore.

(c) Exercise

The more active you are the slimmer you are likely to become. However, rushing around and being busy is unfortunately not the right sort of activity. What you need is the sort of exercise that makes your heart rate rise and induces sweating. Exercise raises your metabolic rate so you need more food as well as burning more food when you are actually working those muscles. In addition, the only way to reshape your body is to build lean tissue. You will want to eat more but don't worry about that; you will still lose fat.

Build up your activity level gradually, following the advice in sections 17.2, 17.6, 17.7 and 17.9.

(d) Strategies for persistent fat problems

Chemicals or other substances that are useless or dangerous to your body are broken down by the liver so that they can be excreted. Our environment is heavily loaded with such substances, and we may take in more through a heavily processed diet and particularly through smoking, drinking alcohol and taking drugs and medicines. So the detoxification capacity of the liver is quite heavily stressed most of the time. When potential toxins arrive faster than the liver can cope with them, it can transfer them into fat. Fat acts as a store for a massive range of chemicals, including drug and pesticide residues, some food additives and preservatives and many industrial chemicals. Shifting this polluted fat is particularly difficult because burning it will release the chemicals it contains and thus stimulate the fat-production response once more. Your body will tend to resist all conventional efforts at weight loss if this is your problem; exercise will make you feel ill, while dieting will drop your metabolic rate and cause excessive tiredness, headaches and other symptoms.

People who suffer from allergies are particularly likely to have a persistent fat problem because their bodies will treat a greater range of substances as toxic. If you fall into this group it is especially important to reduce your exposure to *all* chemicals—household chemicals such as detergents, perfumed products and sprays, household chemicals and solvents, exhaust fumes, smoke, pesticides, food additives, etc.

If you cut your intake of toxic chemicals, and at the same time increase your body's capacity for coping with them, you can overcome this persistent fat-retention problem. A detailed explanation of the approach, with specific information on diet and activity patterns which will produce permanent fat loss, is given in our book *Fat Free Forever*.

(e) Changing perspective

Accepting yourself for what you are is an essential part of a healthy fat-reduction strategy. Looking at yourself naked in a mirror is a valuable exercise; acknowledge what you are rather than struggling to fit some image that perhaps could never be you. People with weight problems often have very distorted images of themselves and this makes their difficulties even greater.

Throw away your bathroom scales! You are not a sack of potatoes and your weight is irrelevant to your condition. You can be "underweight" according to the charts and still be fat; or you can be "overweight" but lean and muscular. Aim for a better *quality* of flesh; the quantity will look after itself if you treat your body properly.

Eating for emotional reasons is very common. If you tend to binge you will discover that your desire to stuff yourself with food when you are alone or unhappy will diminish when you treat yourself with care. Depriving yourself of food because you are anxious about your weight very often leads to bingeing and overeating when willpower flags. And if you have been dieting, overeating will have much more serious effects on your waistline than if you adopt the no-diet strategy described above. Most people find that once they cease to override or punish their bodies and stop depriving themselves of nourishment, they no longer react to emotional anguish with hunger.

If there is an emotional component to your weight problem, read Susie Orbach's *Fat Is a Feminist Issue.* It is a deeply comforting book which contains detailed advice on changing distorted reactions to food.

11

Liver, Kidneys and Bladder

This chapter is concerned with liver and kidney disease, including chronic liver problems, gallstones, kidney stones and kidney failure; it also covers bladder problems including cystitis, bed-wetting and urinary incontinence.

SECTION INDEX

11.1 *The liver, kidneys and bladder*

11.2 *Liver disease*

11.3 *Drugs for liver disease*

11.4 *Dealing with liver problems*

11.5 *Gallbladder inflammation (cholecystitis) and gall-stones*

11.6 *Drugs for gallbladder problems*

11.7 *Alternatives to drugs for gallbladder problems*

11.8 *Kidney disease*

11.9 *Kidney stones*

11.10   *Cystitis*
11.11   *Drugs for cystitis*
11.12   *Alternatives to drugs for cystitis*
11.13   *Bed-wetting and urinary incontinence*
11.14   *Drugs for bed-wetting and urinary incontinence*
11.15   *Alternatives to drugs for bed-wetting*
11.16   *Alternatives to drugs for urinary incontinence*

11.1   THE LIVER, KIDNEYS AND BLADDER

These organs maintain a healthy balance of nutrients and water in the body. The liver transforms food into products that are useful to the cells throughout the body; it stores nutrients and it breaks down unwanted substances so that they can be eliminated. It has many other important functions too, such as temperature control and the regulation of levels of a wide variety of substances in the body. Women have smaller livers than men and are therefore more prone to liver problems.

Attached to the liver is the gallbladder. The gallbladder stores bile acids which are produced by the liver and releases them into the gut for the digestion of fats.

Nutrients and unwanted substances from the liver are attached to special carrier molecules which then circulate in the blood. The nutrients feed the tissues while the waste products are carried to the kidneys where the blood is filtered. Unwanted substances are separated from their carriers and released into urine which is produced by the kidneys using water from the blood. The urine accumulates in the bladder until there is enough to stimulate urination. Finally it is excreted via the urethra, a narrow tube leading out of the body from the bladder.

Problems with these systems can arise from a variety of causes. One of the most important is overload by toxic substances, which can include anything the body identifies as a potential hazard. Precisely what these are can vary from person to person; the body's immune system has the job of identifying what substances may be dangerous, and each person's immune system will have an individual response to any particular one. Allergy occurs when the immune system reacts to harmless substances as if they were poisonous.

The capacity of the liver to deal with poisons is not unlimited, and modern life exposes us to far more chemicals than our bodies were designed to handle. New substances are constantly being developed and released into the environment by the chemical industry. They enter our bodies in the form of pesticide residues and chemical additives in the food we eat; fumes, factory emissions and household chemicals in the air we breathe; chlorine compounds and farming residues in the water we drink; chemicals that penetrate our skin when we use them in cleaning and other everyday activities, and drugs which we take as medicines. Inevitably more and more people are running into problems with toxic substances. They overload the immune system, stress the liver and damage the kidneys. They may be fairly harmless while they are attached to carriers in the blood-stream, but once they are separated from these in the kidneys they are capable of wreaking havoc. The consequences of all this chemical contamination range from immune-system failure, producing vulnerability to infections and allergies, to cancers.

Infection can also be a problem with these crucial organs. Hepatitis (liver inflammation) can be a consequence of viral infection or toxic damage to the liver. Kidney problems, from nephritis to kidney failure, have been linked with infection. In the bladder, the pool of urine can harbor bacteria which cause cystitis.

Our general health depends heavily on the efficient function of these organs. The kidneys must work properly so that the filtration process functions as it should, maintaining a proper balance of water in the body; if this fails, drugs and toxins which are not removed sufficiently quickly and effectively from the blood will accumulate to dangerous levels. In addition essential nutrients and proteins may be lost in the urine. Thus the effects of malfunction in these organs spread throughout the rest of the body.

11.2 LIVER DISEASE

Liver damage is caused by overload with poisons and by infection. The two are linked because toxic stress reduces our defenses against infection. Drugs, solvents, cigarette smoke, pollutants, hormones and the products of tissue breakdown all go through the same process in the liver; when these toxic substances overstretch the liver's coping capacity, the result is damage to its regeneration and internal maintenance processes. The most common single cause of overload in our culture is excessive consumption of alcohol; the all-too-familiar hangover is a symptom of the liver's failure to metabolize alcohol at the rate at which it arrives.

Signs of liver malfunction can be difficult to pin down. Typical symptoms of chronic liver disease include frequent indigestion, nausea, headaches, depression, weakness and a generally run-down feeling. You may also find you react badly to cigarettes and alcohol and you are likely to be highly susceptible to adverse drug reactions. You will probably also lose your appetite and cease to enjoy foods that you used to like.

Acute liver disease, on the other hand, is usually immediately obvious. It causes jaundice which produces a characteristic yellowing of the skin and the whites of the eyes. This develops when bile (produced by the liver from the debris of red blood corpuscles) accumulates in the blood instead of being excreted into the gut. The lack of bile in the gut causes problems with the digestion of fats and makes the stools pale.

11.3   Drugs for liver disease

Liver disease is usually left untreated. Potential damage to the liver by poisons can sometimes be averted by the use of a suitable 'antidote', though this is rare. Chronic liver inflammation is occasionally treated with steroids (see section 6.4(d) for their side-effects).

11.4   Dealing with liver problems

Hangover and short-term toxic stress can be dealt with by immediate activity. If you have been exposed to more alcohol or other poison than you expect your body to be able to handle, go out for a brisk walk or run or dance energetically. *Don't smoke or drink black coffee.* Increase your oxygen use through fairly strenuous movement, lasting at least fifteen minutes and preferably considerably more; this will help the detoxifying enzymes in the liver which need large amounts of oxygen. Avoid the morning-after blues by walking home from the party. Drink plenty of pure water mixed with pure fruit juice.

The liver is capable of healing itself when it gets damaged, so if you have longer-term liver problems you should maximize the conditions for liver health and healing with a diet that provides the specific nutrients required and a life-style that minimizes the demand on your liver until its capacity has improved.

(a) Diet

Your liver breaks down the nutrients in food and removes all the potentially toxic or useless chemicals that you consume with food. The first step to liver health is to reduce the work involved in dealing with food, while at the same time building up its detoxifying capacity. The further you can go towards the sort of diet our ancestors had, the easier the task for your liver. Eat raw food whenever possible, with a fresh salad at least once a day. Don't touch processed or "junk" food. Avoid all synthetic additives. Eat organic food (see section 18.2); this is important not only because it is unsprayed and free from potentially poisonous pesticide residues but because it has a better balance of vitamins and micronutrients. Many nutrients are involved in the metabolic work of the liver, and you cannot afford to go short of these if your liver is to return to fully effective functioning.

Certain nutrients are essential for detoxification; if you are short of these your liver capacity will be reduced. They include the sulphur-containing amino-acids, iron, zinc, B-group vitamins, especially folic acid, and vitamin C (see sections 18.4 and 18.5(a) for sources). Do not rely on supplements: your body may not react to them as it would to natural foods. Further details of a diet and lifestyle regime for promoting liver health are given in our book *Fat Free Forever.*

Eat whenever you feel you want to; do not go hungry. A number of small meals is better than a few large ones. Avoid fried and fatty foods but eat raw vegetable oils such as cold-pressed olive and sunflower oil (excellent in salad dressings) which contain essential nutrients. Unless you know they are organic, avoid all animal products apart from free-range eggs, fish, natural low-fat yogurt and skimmed milk. Animals concentrate pollutants in their fat (including milk fat) and body organs, and these pollutants will put further demand on your liver. (See sections 18.1 and 18.2.)

Drink herb teas, dandelion coffee, bottled or purified water, organic fruit or pure vegetable juices. Always drink enough—don't go thirsty. As far as possible avoid ordinary tea and coffee. Refuse all alcohol and soft drinks.

(b) Smoking

Cigarettes are likely to nauseate you if you have liver problems. But however they make you feel, you should avoid them. Cigarette smoke contains more than 200 different poisons; liver cancer is one of many cancers that are linked with cigarette smoking.

(c) Environment

Many pollutants reach the liver through our skin and lungs, so reducing the level of these in your environment could be important. There are very wide individual differences in sensitivity to chemicals and naturally occurring toxins. As a general rule if a substance gives trouble to other people it will load your liver even if you are not aware of symptoms associated with it. So avoid solvents, smoke, fumes, detergents and household and workplace chemicals. Don't use chemical fly killers, flea sprays or air fresheners. Keep away from chemically contaminated places such as hairdressers, hospitals, dry cleaners, and shoe-repair and paint stores. Don't use glue, polyester resin, or other strong-smelling household products.

More information on harmful chemicals, their sources and how to avoid them is given in Fritsch's *The Household Pollutant Guide* (see Bibliography).

(d) Activity

Physical activity stimulates the liver. Any activity which makes you breathe heavily will increase the oxygen available to the liver and aid detoxification, while longer sessions of fairly strenuous activity will cause the liver to use its energy stores of glycogen. These stores will be regenerated when you eat, so the more you use them the more they will become accessible to you.

When liver damage makes you feel weak and tired, physical activity is the last thing you could imagine enjoying. Just rest and eat well while you recover. But as soon as activity becomes feasible, start moving. Walking in fresh air is very helpful and will improve your health. Breathe slowly and deeply (see section 16.5). Don't try to do any strenuous activity (such as running) until your liver is functioning effectively again. Too much could set you back, giving you headaches and inducing nausea. Build your capacity gently; once your health has returned, use demanding or long-lasting physical exercise to improve your detoxifying capacity and protect you from future liver problems. (See sections 17.5, 17.7 and 17.8.)

11.5 GALLBLADDER INFLAMMATION (CHOLECYSTITIS) AND GALLSTONES

Gallbladder problems are particularly common among women of middle age in Western countries, although other groups also suffer from them. Nobody knows precisely why they develop, but a diet high in animal fats and low in fiber is at least partly to blame. Gallbladder inflammation and infection is usually associated with gallstones; the symptoms are indigestion and pain in the upper abdomen, especially after a meal of fatty foods.

11.6 DRUGS FOR GALLBLADDER PROBLEMS

Infections can be treated with antibiotics (see section 5.7) but they are likely to recur unless the underlying stone problem is sorted out. The liver produces chenodeoxycholic acid, which dissolves gallstones; synthetic forms are now available and are used to treat small stones. Brand names include Chenix and Decholin. Side effects include diarrhea, itching and possible adverse effects on the liver.

11.7 ALTERNATIVES TO DRUGS FOR GALLBLADDER PROBLEMS

The Western processed diet causes gallstones, so recovery from gall-bladder problems and prevention of stone formation requires a reversal of dietary trends. Adopting a high-fiber organic whole-food diet (see sections 18.2 and 18.3) seems to prevent gallstone formation. Cut out all animal fat (see section 18.1), and give up animal produce completely if you can. Vegetarians have much lower rates of gallbladder problems than meat eaters, and among vegans (who eat neither meat nor dairy produce) they are unknown. Get your protein from nuts, beans and whole grains. Give up sugar; it increases the risk of gallstone formation (see section 18.11).

11.8 KIDNEY DISEASE

Like the liver, the kidneys play a crucial part in dealing with potentially poisonous substances that enter our bodies. In the fine tubules of the kidneys, toxins and wastes are removed from the bloodstream. Tiny blood vessels form a delicate network around the tubules, and dissolved wastes are shed through their specialized membranes into urine.

Predictably, problems arise at these membranes. They can be exposed to high levels of poisonous substances, especially if you are taking medicines that must be excreted through the kidneys. We are all aware of the constant outcry about the lack of facilities for treatment of kidney patients, but it begs a crucial question: why are kidneys failing so often? Perhaps the reluctance to question the causes of kidney failure has to do with the fact that medicine—in the form of drug treatment—is a major contributor to it.

Very many poisons are capable of damaging the kidneys. Most drugs can damage both the liver and kidneys if they are taken in larger doses than the body can deal with. The immediate stress of a course of drug therapy is made worse by the chronic stress of everyday exposure to a multiplicity of poisons and synthetic substances that are of no value to the body; the way we eat and live makes us particularly susceptible to kidney damage. As we age, our kidneys gradually become less efficient at filtering toxins and more vulnerable to damage with normal doses of drugs. Kidney failure is increasing among older people, and it is now the tenth most common cause of death.

Infection is the most common reason for kidney failure early in life. It seems that the body's own immune response is involved; antibodies begin to attack the kidneys after being stimulated to fight disease such as throat infections. Antibiotic therapy can add to this problem. Chronic illness such as diabetes can also lead to kidney damage. When the kidneys are already under stress they are more likely to suffer when exposed to other stresses; so all these problems interact with one another.

The best strategy for prolonging the health of your kidneys must therefore be one which promotes a high level of general health. Minimizing exposure to potential poisons is one requirement; eating wisely and well to build resistance to infection and chronic illness is another.

If kidney disease leads to renal failure you may have no alternative but to hope for a transplant and rely on dialysis in the meantime. But before this happens you may be able to reverse the course of the deterioration by careful attention to diet. Adopt an organic whole-food diet (see section 18.2) with the minimum of protein. Avoid all animal products. Eat your food raw whenever possible, and drink plenty of pure bottled water such as Perrier.

11.9 KIDNEY STONES

Kidney stones are usually made of calcium oxalate derived from food. They form when the metabolic balance of the body is disrupted. They may produce no symptoms for years, but if they start to move out of the kidneys they cause excruciating pain and they may block the elimination of urine, leading to further damage. Large stones may need to be removed by surgery; smaller stones may be passed out of the body in the urine, but you will probably need potent pain-relieving drugs to help you through the process.

Oxalates are common in food, particularly rhubarb, tea, chocolate, peanuts, spinach and beetroot, and you would be wise to avoid these if you are prone to stone formation. Calcium in food seems not to affect the process directly, but cutting down on whole milk and cheese is nevertheless a sensible strategy partly because of the high level of pollutants in milk fat and partly because lactose (milk sugar) enhances calcium absorption. Calcium in very hard water can precipitate stone formation, and softening your water may be enough to prevent it; we know of sufferers from kidney stones who have been able to deal with the problem simply by buying a water softener. Although this is not considered relevant by most members of the medical profession (we have been unable to find any reference to it in the clinical literature) it does seem appropriate in view of the chemical composition of the stones.

Stone formation is more common in people who eat a large proportion of protein, especially meat, and relatively little starchy food such as bread. Sugar in the diet also increases the amount of calcium in the urine, and problems with sugar metabolism (notably diabetes) are also implicated. A high-fiber whole-food diet with plenty of fresh fruit, vegetables and grain will help (see section 18.2). Clinical studies have shown that magnesium and vitamin B_6 will prevent stone formation (see sections 18.4(e) and 18.4(l)), as will drinking a lot of water. You should drink enough to keep your urine very pale, if necessary waking during the night for an extra glass of water. This flushes out any tiny crystals before they get large enough to lodge in the kidneys.

Alcohol puts stress on the kidneys, increases the excretion of calcium and has an adverse effect on the metabolism of magnesium and vitamin B_6. Avoid it or drink only in moderation, flushing the alcohol through your system with plenty of water.

11.10 CYSTITIS

Cystitis is an inflammation of the urinary system which can lead to kidney damage if it occurs frequently. It is more common in women. Sufferers feel a frequent and urgent need to urinate, but doing so causes burning pain and there may be little or no urine. Sometimes the urine is bloodstained, and it may contain pus. There may be pain in the lower abdomen and a mild fever.

Cystitis is often assumed to be due to bacterial infection, but research has revealed only the most tenuous of links between symptoms and bacteria. In about 50% of cases no sign of infection can be found, while bacteria are often present in the urine of symptom-free people. When bacteria are involved they tend to be types that are harmlessly present in the healthy body—most often *Escherichia coli*, which lives in the bowel. These organisms are around all the time so it is important to understand what disrupts our healthy relationship with them.

11.11   DRUGS FOR CYSTITIS

Cystitis may be treated with a range of antibiotic drugs. It is sensible to have a urine test before treatment begins because many of the organisms involved are now resistant to common antibiotics. If you consult a doctor about your cystitis, take a urine sample in a clean bottle for testing.

The antibiotics most often prescribed for urinary tract infections are sulphonamides (see section 5.7 (c)). Side effects are relatively common and can be serious, especially in people with impaired kidney function.

Cystitis is sometimes treated with nitrofurantoin (Furadantin, Macrodantin). Adverse effects include nausea, vomiting, rashes, nerve damage, respiratory problems and liver disease. Among the many other antibiotics prescribed for urinary tract infection are ampicillin (section 5.7(a)) and tetracycline (section 5.7(b)).

11.12   ALTERNATIVES TO DRUGS FOR CYSTITIS

Cystitis tends to be a recurring problem but it can be avoided. If you suffer an attack you may be able to cut it short without recourse to medical help.

(a) Avoiding chemical irritation

Chemical irritation due to excessive "hygiene"—use of soaps, deodorants, disinfectants and detergents—will make you more susceptible to cystitis; wearing pantyhose, panties and trousers made of synthetic fibers that do not allow the genital area to breathe compounds the problem, especially in women.

Ensure that only natural fabrics cover your crotch; cotton is best. Change your underwear frequently, washing it with pure soap if possible and rinsing thoroughly in soft water so that no residue is left. Even the smallest quantity of most detergent powders—especially those that contain enzymes—can irritate the delicate openings of the vagina and urethra, making you vulnerable to infection. Do not use them. Also avoid all products which give a "fresh" smell to your clothes.

Never allow any deodorant or perfumed product near your genital area. Bath salts, bubble baths and bath oils are not for you; in fact you would probably be wiser to shower because the soap you use on your body will be in the bathwater and it could irritate the vulva. Don't wash your hair in the bath. Don't use talcum powder or sanitary products that contain "freshening" agents. And don't let your sexual partner introduce soap or any other potential irritant into you on an insufficiently rinsed penis, on dirty or chemically contaminated fingers or in any form of sex play.

(b) Hygiene

Since organisms which live in the bowel can cause cystitis and vaginitis, women should always wipe themselves from front to back after going to the bathroom. This is an important lesson for all little girls, and one which they must never forget.

Genital cleanliness helps to keep cystitis at bay, but it is essential to avoid chemical irritation in your efforts to achieve hygiene. Wash with a shower head or bidet if possible. Never use soap or any other cleansing product; just rinse thoroughly with warm water and pat dry with a soft towel which, like your panties, is kept free from detergent or other chemical contamination.

(c) Diet

Sugary urine provides a favorable environment for any hostile organism. This is one of many reasons for cutting sugar out of your diet (see section 18.11).

All cystitis sufferers should drink more water. Even if you think you are drinking enough, have more. Five pints a day is about right for most people. Avoid strong tea and coffee. Try to avoid alcohol. If you do have it, make sure it is well diluted; choose long drinks, alternate shorts with mineral water and mix your wine with pure water. All this liquid will make you produce copious amounts of dilute urine, which is the effect you are after. Don't delay if you need to urinate, and always empty your bladder completely. Try to squeeze some more out a little while after you think you have finished.

Cystitis can be a symptom of food allergy. To identify any possible dietary culprit, keep a diary of your cystitis attacks and a record of everything you eat. You may be able to pick up a recurring pattern. (See section 18.8.)

(d) Sex

Sex is often a problem for cystitis sufferers. For some women, symptoms begin only after they become sexually active, or they may follow unusually vigorous sexual activity. Women can minimize damage to delicate tissues by ensuring adequate lubrication; don't hesitate to use K-Y jelly (*not* Vaseline or skin cream) if necessary. Don't have intercourse with a full bladder, and always urinate immediately afterward to flush out any bacteria that may have made their way into your urethra during intercourse. Then wash carefully in cool water; dissolve a tablespoon of sea salt in the water to soothe any tenderness.

Sex or relationship problems can also play a part in precipitating cystitis. Like other forms of illness linked with sexual activity, it can emerge as an unconscious way of avoiding conflicts associated with sex. In addition the vaginal bruising that often precipitates cystitis in women is more likely if you are not completely aroused. This may have an emotional basis or it could reflect poor sexual technique. If you suspect that your cystitis is associated with problems in sexual relationships, a counselor will help you sort them out.

Cystitis has been found to be particularly common in chronically anxious people. Dealing with the source of the problem is likely to have the best results.

(e) Coping with an attack of cystitis

Act fast! As soon as you feel the merest suspicion of symptoms, start drinking. Dissolve a teaspoonful of bicarbonate in a pint of water and drink it without delay; it will make your urine alkaline and discourage bacteria. Then drink a cup of strong coffee to encourage rapid urine production. Drink another half pint of water half an hour later. Repeat the sequence hourly three times. With luck this prompt action will abort the attack. Keep bicarbonate at work if you are prone to attacks there. If your blood pressure tends to be high, substitute potassium citrate for bicarbonate. Hot-water bottles on the lower belly or between the thighs, or a hot bath (no soap!), will help soothe pain.

Take a specimen of urine early in the attack to give to your doctor if necessary. If your symptoms persist, and especially if you feel feverish, with pain in the lower back, or if there is blood or pus in your urine, you should see a doctor; infection can spread to the kidneys and you may need antibiotic treatment. Take your urine sample when you consult.

Support for cystitis sufferers is available from the Interstitial Cystitis Association, P.O. Box 1553, Madison Square Station, New York, NY 10159.

11.13　BED-WETTING AND URINARY INCONTINENCE

Bed-wetting and incontinence occur when people—usually the young or old—do not receive sufficient warning stimuli from the bladder to tell them that they need to urinate. With children the problem is likely to sort itself out in time; with adults it has a range of different causes, including temporary illness, loss of tone in the pelvic muscles after childbirth, injury or disease of the spinal cord, and local conditions affecting the bladder and nearby organs.

11.14 DRUGS FOR BED-WETTING AND URINARY INCONTINENCE

These drugs act on the nervous system to make the bladder muscle less reactive. Anticholinergic drugs such as propantheline (Pro-Banthine) may be prescribed; difficulty with urination, an unwanted side effect when these drugs are used in other contexts such as ulcer therapy, is the desired effect in this case. Other adverse effects such as dry mouth, blurred vision, disturbances of heartbeat and more rarely the eye disease glaucoma remain unwanted. Anticholinergic drugs are described in section 8.6 (*a*).

11.15 ALTERNATIVES TO DRUGS FOR BED-WETTING

Bed-wetting is much more common than some parents realize: 20% of three-year-olds, 10% of five-year-olds and 5% of eleven-year-olds wet their beds. Your child may be a particularly deep sleeper and take longer learning to wake than most others. There is usually no cause to worry; abnormalities leading to bed-wetting are very rare.

Nevertheless, it is a nuisance and an embarrassment, and if your child is over three it is time to act to prevent it. Limit fluid intake in the hours before bed. Don't refuse your child a drink, but keep the quantities small. Encourage drinking early in the day. Don't give your child tea, coffee or soft drinks (especially colas) because these are diuretics and will increase the production of urine. Stick to fruit juices and water. Lift the child out of bed when you retire and sit him or her on the potty. Most children will go back to sleep very quickly afterward.

If the bed-wetting has started recently in a child who has been dry, the most probable cause is emotional stress. Starting school or the birth of a new brother or sister could be responsible. If you suspect such a cause, do all you can to reassure your child; take him or her for a relaxing walk before bed; and be confident that the bed-wetting problem will be resolved again before long.

Children can be trained to wake up before wetting the bed with gadgets that wake them with a bell or buzzer as soon as the first drops of moisture fall on the sheet. After a while they learn to anticipate the bell in much the same way as we learn to wake just before an alarm goes off. These can be obtained through school health services and doctors.

11.16   ALTERNATIVES TO DRUGS FOR URINARY INCONTINENCE

(a) Drug-induced incontinence

Sometimes incontinence is precipitated by the use of diuretic drugs which increase the volume of urine. (See section 9.10(b) for information about diuretics). If it is possible to avoid them, the incontinence problem may be solved.

Some common drinks have diuretic effects, so you could try avoiding these for a trial period of a couple of weeks. They are tea, coffee, cola drinks and alcohol. Use substitutes such as herb teas, dandelion coffee and fruit juice. Restricting the quantity you drink is likely to be helpful if you are an avid tea or coffee drinker and habitually consume many cups a day. Change to pure water, drink only when you are thirsty and only until your thirst is quenched. You will want to drink much less.

Sedatives and tranquilizing drugs can cause confusion and drowsiness which result in incontinence. If you are taking any tablets to help you sleep, try to wean yourself off them; this could be enough to allow you to regain bladder control. (See section 4.10 for advice on sleeping.)

(b) Stress incontinence

This problem is particularly common in women who have borne children, affecting about one woman in three at some time in her life. Urine leaks out with slight exertion—a cough or a sneeze—because the muscles around the bladder neck and in the pelvic floor are overstretched and weak. If no action is taken to strengthen these muscles the problem can get gradually worse. The exercises that follow should be carried out for at least three months, a dozen times each day. Improvement will be gradual so you must persevere.

1. Sit, stand or lie comfortably without tensing your abdomen, behind or leg muscles and pretend you are trying to control diarrhea by tightening the ring of muscle around the anus. Do this repeatedly.
2. Sit on the toilet and begin to urinate. While doing so, try to stop the flow in midstream by contracting the muscles around the urethra. Repeat the exercise until you feel totally sure of the movement and of the sensation of applying conscious control.
3. Sit, stand or lie and practice tightening first the anal muscles, then those around the urethra, then both together. Count to four slowly, then release. Repeat four times, hourly if possible.

These exercises can become habitual; you can do them while watching TV, lying in bed, standing at the bus stop or talking to the minister. The more you do them the stronger the muscles will become.

(c) Urgency

In some cases the urge to pass urine is followed almost immediately by leakage unless the bladder is emptied at once. If this condition occurs suddenly it may be due to infection or other bladder irritation and you should consult your doctor. In elderly people the onset is usually gradual and has no serious pathological implications.

First, it makes sense to acknowledge the problem. Make sure you don't have to go far or struggle upstairs to get to a bathroom. A commode in your living room may be the answer. Empty your bladder completely with each urination; bending forward at the waist will help. After you have emptied your bladder, wait a minute before leaving the toilet and see if you can't produce a little more. Pass urine at two-hour intervals whether or not you feel the need to do so. The bladder can be trained to respond to this routine. Set a kitchen timer or alarm clock to remind you to use the bathroom at these regular intervals. If your bladder needs emptying more often than this, practice stopping and restarting the flow every time you urinate in order to strengthen the muscles. Use this method to hold on to the urine for slightly longer before passing urine next time. Day by day, you will be able to extend the period of time before you have to urinate, and in time you will find you can last long enough to use the two-hour routine.

Avoid constipation; a full bowel will put pressure on the bladder. See section 8.16 for advice if you ever suffer from it.

Choose clothes which allow quick and easy use of the bathroom. Full skirts or wraparound styles worn with crotchless tights or long socks are sensible for women; men can get specially designed quick-opening trousers.

Help, information and support for incontinent people and their families is offered by the Simon Foundation, Box 815, Wilmette, IL 60091, (312) 864–3913, and by Help for Incontinent People, P.O. Box 544, Union, SC 29379, (803) 585–8780.

12

Pain

In this chapter we shall be considering alternatives to drugs for the relief of chronic and acute pain, and specific alternatives for headache (including migraine) and back pain.

SECTION INDEX

12.1   How we experience pain
12.2   Drugs for minor pains
12.3   Alternatives to drugs for minor pains
12.4   Tension headache
12.5   Migraine headache
12.6   Drugs for migraine
12.7   Alternatives to drugs for migraine
12.8   Other types of headache
12.9   Chronic pain
12.10   Drugs for the relief of chronic pain
12.11   Alternatives to drugs for chronic pain
12.12   Back pain

12.1 HOW WE EXPERIENCE PAIN

The sensation of pain is transmitted along specialized nerve fibers from the site of the pain to the brain, where the experience is perceived and our reactions are directed. At first this seems like a straightforward situation, but research and clinical experience have proved that it is not. The sensation of pain is affected by systems that are little understood. We know, for example, that it is possible to feel pain in a limb that has been amputated (phantom limb pain), and also that many pain victims show no sign of damage that can explain their feelings. There is no straightforward relationship between tissue damage, injury or disease and the experience of pain.

The medical approach to pain relief concentrates on the physiology of pain, on the circuits that connect painful parts to the brain. If the cause of the pain can be identified it is often possible to interrupt the circuit with drugs or surgery and thus relieve the pain. But while medical and surgical approaches can be very successful with acute pain, especially when due to injury, they often fail with chronic pain. People with conditions such as long-established back pain may go through repeated surgery and take increasing doses of drugs which become less and less effective as time goes on. Some sufferers face additional problems because in the absence of any evidence of physical damage to any part of the body, they may be treated as though their pain were nonexistent, imaginary or "neurotic." They experience not only the distress of the pain but also rejection by a medical system that fails to acknowledge it as a real problem.

Recently, however, great advances have been made in our knowledge of the psychology of pain. Instead of concentrating on the "hardware" of the body, psychologists have been studying the "software." As a consequence a whole series of strategies has been developed which, used together, have transformed the lives of many chronic pain sufferers. The key to this approach is the realization that the *perception* of pain is determined by nerve circuits that can be programed—or "conditioned"—to be highly sensitive to any possible pain or to be relatively insensitive. This process of conditioning begins in infancy; without being aware of it we actually teach our children to experience pain.

Pain prevention begins in childhood; parents have a responsibility to ensure that their children do not grow up in such a way that they are liable to experience high levels of pain. The secret is to appear stoical in the presence of children, to play down the severity of any pain and to avoid complaining about it. Teach by example that suffering should be ignored as far as possible, and pay as little attention as you can to children's pain. Try to assess the seriousness of any injury quietly and calmly; when adults panic, they make it much worse for the child and teach the child to fear it more. Don't worry if you appear hard-hearted; in the long term it is a greater kindness to dismiss your child's distress (while attending to any injury, naturally) than to show excessive concern about it.

When we experience pain we normally communicate it to those around us by complaining, moaning, grimacing, limping and a whole range of other cues which psychologists call pain behaviors. Our companions will usually respond with concern, paying greater attention to us than otherwise. If we are injured or suddenly seriously ill this is clearly beneficial, but if there is nothing that others can do to relieve our pain it can become harmful because we learn that showing pain brings attention and caring. If we want more attention than we normally get, we may begin to experience more pain in order to elicit it. This does not happen at a conscious level. It is part of the process of conditioning, a type of learning that happens without awareness. Conditioning affects involuntary reactions and experiences, and pain can be conditioned all too readily. When this happens the pain is liable to persist and even increase in severity in the absence of any physiological abnormality.

The psychological approach to pain relief involves reversing this conditioning cycle. Just as the experience of pain develops through a type of learning, so we can deliberately set about learning another set of reactions designed to minimize pain. This is, admittedly, a slow process and one that demands a high level of motivation in the sufferer; but it is one that is being successfully used in an increasing number of pain clinics and which offers lasting relief to people who have tried every other approach without real benefit.

Conditioning is just one of many psychological modulators of pain. Expectations, fear, depression and tension also affect the amount of pain we feel. Pain sufferers should therefore read chapters

4 and 16 and work through the advice given for stress and depression even if they are not aware of such problems.

12.2 Drugs for minor pains

Over-the-counter analgesics are generally taken for minor, relatively short-lived types of pain such as headache. They are based on three drugs: acetaminophen, aspirin and ibuprofen. There are many brand names, and special claims are made for some of them, but the unbranded forms (e.g., soluble aspirin) are just as effective and much cheaper.

These products have relatively few side effects (see section 5.3 for details) and are usually safe in short-term use, although they can be hazardous if taken frequently for a period of years. All can kill in overdose. Acetaminophen is particularly nasty because it damages the liver; this may not be apparent for a day or two after the overdose, but it can cause a miserable and irreversible illness which ends in death after a period of days or weeks.

Aspirin is the most useful of the over-the-counter analgesics for most forms of pain; it reduces fever and inflammation as well as relieving pain. However, if you suffer from stomach ulcers or any tendency to bleeding from the stomach or intestine, it can be very dangerous and should be totally avoided. Pregnant women and people who use tablets for diabetes should avoid aspirin. Asthmatics should be aware that sensitivity to aspirin can precipitate asthma attacks. Ibuprofen is chemically similar to aspirin; if you cannot take aspirin, ibuprofen is likely to be just as bad for you.

No medicine containing aspirin should ever be given to children running a fever; aspirin is believed to cause a serious illness called Reye's syndrome which can be fatal. This syndrome seems to develop only after virus infection in children.

12.3 Alternatives to drugs for minor pains

The most common type of minor pain is headache, for which we give more specific advice in sections 12.4 through 12.8. If you suffer from menstrual pain read section 14.7 in addition to the material here.

There are two main approaches to the reduction of pain perception. One involves adjusting one's mental focus, while the other relies on blocking pain sensation through the use of competing forms of stimulation.

Mental pain reduction should begin if possible before the pain occurs. If you are going to have to go through a potentially painful experience you should first work on your expectations. Do not anticipate the worst; deliberately stop yourself from imagining that the pain will be more than slight. If you are accompanying someone else to an appointment with a dentist or other source of potential pain, play down the possibility that they will get hurt. Research has repeatedly shown that those who expect severe pain will feel it much more intensely than those who expect it to be minor. Films in which patients show little distress as they undergo dental treatment, injections or minor surgery have a pain-reducing effect on people who are about to undergo the same treatment, while films in which patients show marked distress under similar circumstances intensify the pain. It is important, therefore, that parents and others responsible for children should try to ensure that they are exposed only to models who react well to pain. The effect this will have on the child's anticipation of pain will be most effective if the model is similar in age and other characteristics.

When pain does occur its intensity can be reduced by a deliberate effort to shift your mental focus away from it. Don't think about it; think about something else, preferably something pleasant or a puzzle that will occupy your mind as completely as possible. Dentists have discovered that distraction from pain can be useful; many now have radios playing and interesting pictures on the walls or ceiling where their patients can focus on them. Whether you listen to music or read a gripping book, make a clay pot or watch a good film, the important thing is that your attention should be on something other than your pain.

Muscular tension intensifies pain, so use the relaxation routines described in section 16.11 or bring your own personal relaxation system into play to reduce your experience of pain. Deep relaxation is sometimes enough to stop pain completely. Methods of this type, which are particularly highly developed among yogis and fakirs in India, can be used to permit amazing feats of endurance or exposure to hazards without injury or pain.

Competing stimulation of a physical nature is also valuable for pain relief. Psychologist Professor Ron Melzack and physiologist Patrick Wall have shown how sensory input can completely block the perception of pain. They have proposed the existence of a "pain gate" within the brain which can actually be shut by stimulation. The most effective type of stimulation seems to vary with the pain. Heat, cold, vibration, electrical stimulation and rubbing can all reduce pain. Try a hot-water bottle or a bag of frozen peas on the painful area, stimulate it with a massager or use a transcutaneous nerve stimulator (see section 12.11(f)).

If you experience repeated painful episodes from one part of the body get a book on acupressure (shiatsu) and find out which point you can rub for an analgesic effect. Chinese acupuncturists have discovered links between particular points on the body and organs or areas which experience analgesia when these points are stimulated. How this works is unclear, but experiments in both the clinic and the laboratory have demonstrated unequivocally that it does work. While professional stimulation with acupuncture needles (see chapter 2) is undoubtedly more effective than simple rubbing, it is still true that you can achieve significant analgesia using this method without any equipment.

Finally, stimulation can come from muscular movement. Choose a form of movement that does not involve the painful part directly. Depending on the site of your pain, cycling or rowing or sanding down a piece of furniture could have surprising analgesic effects, while sex can be the best painkiller of all. The harder you work at your chosen form of activity, the greater the pain relief you are likely to experience. If you really get going so that you are panting with effort you may find that the surge of painkilling chemicals in the brain that accompanies physical effort is enough to overcome your problem completely.

12.4 TENSION HEADACHE

Headache is probably the most common pain we experience, and there are some quite specific ways to deal with it. There are many forms and causes; we shall subdivide them into tension headache (the most common form), migraine headache (sections 12.5 through 12.7) and an assortment of other headaches (section 12.8).

Headache produced by tension in the neck muscles is felt in the top of the head (perhaps as though a band had been tightened around the head), in the forehead or behind the eyes. This type of headache can occur at any time, though it is more common in the afternoon, and it can recur day after day. If you suffer from it frequently, you need to deal with the root causes of the stress that you are under. Read chapter 16 and build more relaxation into your life. Counseling may help you to resolve conflicts. Relaxation exercises will help you to relax those neck muscles, and physical activity, especially swimming, will also be beneficial. You may find that the answer is just to have more time to yourself when you can lie back and doze undisturbed.

There are a number of specific remedies for the relief of headache once it has developed. Massage is one; see if you can persuade a friend or partner to knead the muscles at the back of the neck and around the shoulders. This may be sufficient to relieve the pain. If you don't have a masseuse you can call upon, take a walk outdoors. Concentrate on making yourself as tall as possible; imagine that your head is suspended from the sky by a fine string attached to the top of the crown and let this imaginary string gently pull you upward. At the same time deliberately relax your shoulders, but make sure they fall back, not forward. Breathe slowly and deeply as you walk, telling yourself that you are eliminating tension with each exhalation.

Poor posture makes tension headaches worse. If you work at a desk or keyboard, check that your chair is the right height so that you are not holding yourself more stiffly than you need. Check too that you are not squinting or tensing yourself to avoid glare; tinted glasses can help to prevent headaches. Finally, get up at intervals to shake yourself out; try to avoid getting too fixed in a position that may involve tension in the neck. Frequent movement and short breaks will also improve your efficiency, so it makes sense to do this.

Suppressed emotions—anger, frustration, fear—often cause tension in neck and head muscles. If you tend to keep your feelings to yourself, see if you can be a little more assertive and loosen up verbally, telling people more often and more honestly how you feel. You may find that your headaches disappear when you allow your emotions a freer rein. If you find it very difficult to admit your feelings, consult a counselor or psychologist; you may need help in this area in order to become free of your headaches.

12.5   MIGRAINE HEADACHE

Migraine headaches are distinguished from tension headaches by a combination of specific characteristics. An "aura" may precede the migraine; this is a highly variable individual experience which can include flashing or jagged light patterns, visual problems, other sensory illusions and mood changes. Migraine pain normally affects only one side of the head, and it is accompanied by nausea and sometimes vomiting. Each migraine sufferer comes to recognize an individual pattern of symptoms which will include some but not necessarily all of these. The problem usually develops in the teenage years and recedes in middle age.

12.6   DRUGS FOR MIGRAINE

Migraine can be treated with a range of different drugs. Most sufferers rely on minor analgesics such as aspirin to ameliorate the worst of the pain during an attack, but specific remedies, mainly based on ergotamine, may be prescribed. Some of these contain an anti-emetic to reduce nausea and suppress vomiting. However, ergotamine is a highly toxic drug which is itself capable of inducing migraine, so sufferers may instead be prescribed minor analgesics in combination with anti-emetics.

(a) Analgesics

Original Formula Midol and Maximum Strength Midol contain aspirin plus an anti-emetic. See section 5.3 for more details about aspirin. The anti-emetic is a type of antihistamine (section 6.4 (a)).

(b) Ergotamine and related drugs

Migraine products often contain ergotamine tartrate in combination with other drugs such as analgesics and belladonna (an anticholinergic drug used to prevent vomiting; see section 8.6 (a)). Examples include Bellergal-S, Cafergot, Ergomar and Wigraine. Isometheptene mucate (Isocom, Midrin, Migralam) is chemically related to ergotamine; Midrin and Migralam also contain acetaminophen.

Ergotamine is given to people who seem not to respond to the safer analgesics. Its side effects include nausea, abdominal pain, muscular cramps, headache and problems with circulation in fingers and toes which may progress to gangrene with chronic overuse. It is particularly hazardous for people with heart or circulatory disease and liver or kidney problems.

(c) Drugs used for migraine prevention

If you suffer frequent migraine headaches you may be given a drug to prevent them. If your doctor thinks your migraine is associated with depression or tension he is likely to prescribe an antidepressant (see section 4.3) or a tranquilizer (section 4.6). Beta blockers (section 9.3(a)) may also be used to prevent migraine. Other products sometimes prescribed for migraine prevention (prophylaxis) include clonidine (Catapres) (see section 9.10(c:2)) and methysergide (Sansert). Methysergide is very dangerous; it can damage the valves of the heart and cause fibrosis of internal organs.

12.7 ALTERNATIVES TO DRUGS FOR MIGRAINE

Like tension headache, migraine is very often stress-related, and it often occurs when severe pressure lifts—at the beginning of holidays or weekends, at the end of exams or after the completion of a vital task. Chronic, long-term stress or conflict can cause severe, apparently intractable migraine. Relaxation therapy has been shown to result in less frequent and less severe attacks for the majority of sufferers. If you suspect your problem could be stress-related, read chapter 16 for advice.

However, migraine can be precipitated by a wide range of other triggers. Your migraine could be caused by one or more of the following: changes in daily routine, skipping meals, sleep (too little or too much), excitement and any strong emotion, stress, unaccustomed effort, especially anaerobic exercise such as weight training, loud or persistent noise, bright flickering light, hormones (including oral contraceptives), working with a VDT (e.g., a computer monitor screen) or watching a television with a poor picture. Certain foods can precipitate attacks, and those most often blamed are chocolate, cheese and other dairy produce (especially mature or blue cheeses), alcohol (especially red wine), citrus fruit, tea and coffee, seafood and fava or broad beans.

If you take oral contraceptives you should change to a nondrug method of birth control. Migraine sufferers may be at particular risk from these and other sex hormones because their blood vessels are abnormally sensitive to the effects of these drugs.

To discover your trigger you will need to keep a diary. When you suffer an attack, make a note of everything you ate or drank in the previous twenty-four hours. Make a note also of any possibly stressful events and of your activities in the preceding day. A pattern is likely to emerge which will allow you to avoid the sort of situation that induces your migraine.

Migraine sufferers can minimize their problem by avoiding flickering lights and wearing polarized sunglasses in bright sun. Simple actions such as crossing the road to avoid a fence that produces a sharp pattern of light and dark can be enough to prevent the onset of migraine. Avoid watching TV when you feel you are on the edge of migraine. If your TV flickers, replace it. If light starts to bother you at all, put on your sunglasses even if you are indoors.

Don't miss meals and don't start strenuous activity without building up to it gradually. Migraine can be a penalty for attempts at rapid weight loss. If your migraine is associated with premenstrual syndrome, take action to achieve a better hormone balance (see chapter 14).

If an attack strikes despite your precautions, this is what you should do. First, take it seriously and act without delay. You should not work, read or drive until you are better; if you do, the attack could last much longer and be more severe than it need be. If you are going to use analgesics, take them immediately. Retire to a dark room and lie down with a couple of pillows under your head. Have a hot drink if you like, but avoid strong tea, coffee, chocolate and instant soups. Use a cold compress (a bag of frozen peas is good) on the site of the pain. Relax as much as possible and try to sleep; the pain will probably go away during sleep.

12.8 OTHER TYPES OF HEADACHE

Headaches can result from the toxic effects of a wide variety of substances, from hunger, infection, overexposure to hot sun or from very cold food or drink. Serious causes of headache such as brain tumor are extremely rare and you should eliminate more common causes that you can deal with yourself before having your headaches investigated further. Toxic headaches include hangovers and headaches due to reaction to drugs and chemicals or pollutants to which you are particularly sensitive. Dieters' and exercisers' headaches may be due to the release of toxic residues as body fat is metabolized (see section 10.8 (d)).

Time will take care of these headaches, but there are steps you can take to reduce your misery. The earlier you act, the better; if you know you have been exposed to too much alcohol, or fumes or other chemicals that tend to give you headaches, take action before the discomfort begins. Spend half an hour in vigorous physical activity such as dancing or brisk walking; do it until you have been breathing heavily for some time and you are quite warm. Activity and deep breathing will increase the level of oxygen in your system and fire up your liver so that it can deal as effectively as possible with poisons. Hangovers can often be avoided completely in this way. Drink plenty of pure water or fruit juice. Recovery may be quicker if you have something to eat. Eggs are particularly good, though you don't need to follow tradition by having them raw! Bland foods such as oatmeal and yogurt are often helpful.

If your diet or exercise regime gives you headaches, change to a detoxifying regime such as the one given in our book *Fat Free Forever*.

Other substances which can cause headaches include the flavor-enhancing food additive monosodium glutamate (MSG). Chinese foods and processed foods are often particularly rich in this substance. If you are fond of eating Chinese food or you go for "junk" or fast food, you could solve your problem by changing to unprocessed whole foods (see sections 18.2 and 18.10).

Headache can be one of the many symptoms of food allergy. You may find that your headaches follow meals or are associated with particular foods. This happens when your body reacts as though those foods were toxic to you. The best way of dealing with this problem is to eliminate the culprits from your diet once you have identified them (see section 18.8).

Another likely cause of headaches is dehydration, especially when associated with stress. If you find your head often aches when you spend a day traveling or rushing around town, try drinking a lot more water. Buy bottles of spring water and drink frequently. If you drink alcohol or strong coffee you will need to balance these with yet more water. You may find that this is enough to prevent these headaches.

12.9 CHRONIC PAIN

There are many causes of chronic pain. Injuries to the back are probably the most common, but problems in any part of the nervous system can result in intractable pain. Often it may not be possible to pinpoint the cause precisely, and even if it is there may be little that conventional medicine can do about it. Surgical attempts at the relief of chronic pain frequently fail and can be very risky.

Long-term pain is different from acute pain and it often requires a completely different type of management. The sort of strategies which are particularly helpful may be the opposite of those used for acute pain. For example, acute injury is often best treated by rest because this allows the damaged tissues to recover; but rest may actually make chronic pain worse and it is generally better to be as active as possible in spite of it.

Drug therapy for chronic pain presents problems that rarely arise with short-term illness. Any pain-reducing drug, when taken day after day for years together, will have diminishing effects. Gradually the dose has to be increased, or more powerful drugs used, to produce the same level of relief. This means that toxicity problems inevitably increase. Sufferers therefore need to learn how to minimize their experience of pain in order to keep the use of drugs as low as possible and to extend their effectiveness. In some cases a combination of nondrug strategies can reduce the need for pain relief to the point where medication is rarely needed.

12.10 DRUGS FOR THE RELIEF OF CHRONIC PAIN

The drugs most frequently used for chronic painful conditions are called nonsteroidal anti-inflammatories (NSAIs).

(a) Aspirin and closely related drugs

See list in section 5.3(b). Aspirin preparations prescribed for chronic pain may contain higher doses than those bought over the counter. To reduce the problem of stomach damage, some products (e.g., Ecotrin Enteric Coated Aspirin) have special coatings and some (e.g., Bufferin) contain chemicals which reduce acidity. Some aspirin preparations are sold especially for chronic painful conditions such as arthritis (e.g., Arthritis Pain Formula, Cama Arthritis Pain Reliever, Momentum Muscular Backache Formula). The pain-relieving drug in these products is ordinary aspirin; their special virtues are in packaging, not potency.

Aspirin reduces inflammation and blocks the effects of certain chemicals (prostaglandins) within the body that are involved in pain production. The side effects of aspirin become significant when it is used in high doses on a regular basis. These include stomach pain, ulceration, bleeding, nausea, hearing disturbances sometimes leading to deafness, vertigo, confusion, allergic reactions and rarely, blood disease. (See also section 5.3.)

(b) Other nonsteroidal anti-inflammatory drugs

Diflunisal (Dolobid); ibuprofen (Advil, Medipren, Midol 200, Motrin, Nuprin, Rufen); indomethacin (Indocin); ketoprofen (Orudis); mefenamic acid (Ponstel); naproxen (Anaprox, Naprosyn); phenylbutazone (Butazolidin); piroxicam (Feldene); sulindac (Clinoril); tolmetin (Tolectin).

These drugs are most likely to be prescribed for arthritis and rheumatism (see chapter 13), but they may be used for many types of chronic painful conditions. Most of them differ from one another primarily in individual patient response; one may be more effective or produce fewer side effects than another. They are liable to cause rashes and/or stomach problems (including nausea, pain, bleeding and ulceration), but the frequency with which these side effects occur varies widely. Other adverse effects associated with some of them include oversensitivity to sunshine, headache, allergic problems and rarely, blood disease. Phenylbutazone has serious and sometimes fatal side effects, particularly blood disorders and severe skin disease; it should be prescribed only in the hospital, and then only for ankylosing spondylitis.

(c) Propoxyphene

Darvon, Darvocet-N, Dolene, Lorcet, Wygesic.

Propoxyphene is a controversial drug. Although it is very widely prescribed, clinical trials have repeatedly failed to demonstrate that it is any better for pain relief than aspirin or acetaminophen—which are both safer and cheaper. Public interest groups, notably the Washington-based Public Citizen Health Research Group, have campaigned for years for the withdrawal of this drug on the grounds that it has been responsible for thousands of accidental-overdose deaths. Propoxyphene is also addictive—which may partly explain its popularity. Propoxyphene products may contain a cocktail of other analgesic drugs; most include acetaminophen; Darvon contains aspirin.

12.11 ALTERNATIVES TO DRUGS FOR CHRONIC PAIN

Learning to live in a way that minimizes pain could mean questioning many of your old habits. It will involve doing things that confront your pain, and which you may have stopped doing because of it. If you follow the strategy outlined below, you can make yourself feel considerably better. This strategy is multifaceted, and you will get maximum benefit if you work on all aspects of it every day. You will need to enlist the help of your family and those who care for you, for their behavior affects the pain you feel. Explain what you are doing and make sure they understand the part they play.

(a) Relaxation

Relaxation will reduce the intensity of your pain and help you to sleep. See sections 16.6 and 16.11 for relaxation techniques and section 4.10 for advice on overcoming sleep problems.

(b) Activity

You should aim to increase your level of activity steadily. Try to take a walk twice a day and go a little further each time. Return to activities that you may have given up because of your pain. You may object that this increases the pain, and in the short term it may if you have become unused to using your muscles and you are weak and stiff. But when pain has continued for several months, movement is not likely to cause any damage; on the contrary, it will promote recovery.

The more vigorous activity you are able to do, the less pain you will feel. If you can do something that really makes demands on your body (hard cycling or swimming, perhaps), your brain will actually begin to release natural pain-reducing chemicals called beta-endorphins that will make you feel better. Exercise will also stimulate your system to produce a pattern of hormones which promote relaxation and healing when the demand on your system is over. Naturally you should not overdo it, but if you build up very gradually, day by day, you will come to know what you can do and what would be too much. Just push yourself a little further each time so that you make steady progress; ignore your regular pain, if it is still with you, but pay attention to any new pain. You are not entering into a regime of self-punishment, nor attempting to prove that activity is dangerous. It is only harmful if you choose to misunderstand messages from your body. (Chapter 17 gives detailed advice on activity.)

If you can go to work or take up a voluntary job, do so. The more you act like a person who is well, the more you will feel well. Ignore any pain you feel and carry on with the job. You will find that you feel less pain as time goes on. Whenever you do things that challenge it you diminish the pain you experience.

(c) Identifying hidden causes

Sometimes the chronic-pain sufferer's problem is associated with other problems for which pain provides a sort of an answer. For example, a man who hates his job but feels he must continue doing it in order to support his family may find that pain gives him a way out of this dilemma. While he is in pain he is not expected to work and cannot be accused of irresponsibility. Similarly, a woman who does not enjoy sex with her husband but who feels guilty about refusing him may develop a pain problem that makes sex impossible. Cases like these are frequently encountered by pain therapists; the pain is real enough for the sufferers, but the cure lies in dealing with the underlying unhappiness rather than in any physical treatment. Every chronic-pain sufferer should try to look closely and calmly at his or her life to find out whether the pain is answering any hidden need and whether the problem could be solved in some other way. If you can separate any such problem from the pain—through being honest about yourself, perhaps with the help of a counselor—then your pain could diminish substantially.

Some rewards for pain are built into our culture, and while they may ease the problems of people with acute pain they can add to the chronic sufferer's burden. Psychologists have demonstrated that rewards can increase both the occurrence and the intensity of pain; the pain victim is actually trained to produce more of it! This is not a voluntary process; it is a consequence of the way the nervous system works. But once you are aware of it, you can start to make deliberate efforts to break the cycle.

The rewards in this context are social. If you show signs of pain— through moaning, grimacing, limping, weeping or complaining— the solicitous people around you will respond with sympathy and attention. Unless they are exceptionally hard-hearted, or they have some knowledge of clinical or behaviorist psychology, they will do their best to make you feel better. They will demand less of you, try to do things for you and help you if they can. In contrast, consider what happens if you are totally stoical. You show no sign of pain so your pain brings nothing from anyone—no attention, no concern. You are left to suffer alone and manage as well as if you had no pain.

Naturally most of us show our pain and elicit the concern of others. At first it seems that we have a lot to lose by behaving in any other way, but we do not realize that we pay for that concern with an increased burden of pain; the attention we enjoy conditions us to show more pain; research in pain clinics has shown that those who show more pain really do experience more. We are aware of the way our feelings determine our actions, but we also need to understand that our actions—and others' reactions to them—play a large part in determining the way we feel. In order to feel less pain we have to *act* as though we feel less pain, and those around us must encourage and reward pain-free or pain-denying behavior. That way the pain we feel will tend to diminish.

(d) Positive thinking

You should try to avoid thinking about your pain; concentrate instead on what you want to do and how you are going to do it. Distract yourself from pain by turning your attention to something else, ideally something that makes you feel cheerful or optimistic. Work through the strategies that you are setting in motion to improve your life; think about the things you are achieving or that you are about to achieve. Ignore completely anything that you have had to give up;

there is nothing to gain by regretting the things you can't do, though with determination you may find you are able to do them and more.

Do not let fear of pain prevent you from doing what you want to do. Focus your mind on what you want to achieve, and remind yourself that humans are able to overcome the most horrendous problems if they really want to. You may think that the man who ran for two days cross country on a broken ankle was an absolute fool, but you cannot ignore the possibilities such feats open up for those who are afraid of doing much less demanding things. It is very much a question of motivation; keep yours up by telling yourself that life is going to be very much better.

You may have had cause for despair if you thought that pain and higher and higher doses of medication were your lot for life, but they are not. Using pain-relieving methods that do not require drugs or surgery—just the power of your mind—you can open up tremendous new opportunities. It is up to you to heal yourself—and it does not require anything more than the mind which every person has. When you concentrate on your abilities instead of on your disabilities, your prospects immediately look less bleak. This is the power of positive thinking; it gets you going when you are tempted to flag.

Fighting chronic pain can be demanding. You will have to make considerable mental effort and you will have to practice before you can keep it up for long. But if you can enlist the help of the people around you in your pain-control strategy, they may be able to maintain a positive course even when you can't.

If you are looking after someone who suffers from chronic pain, you should make attention and concern contingent on *lack* of evidence of pain. This means that you should turn away when the sufferer grimaces or complains of pain; you should ignore pain whenever possible. Obviously, you need to use this strategy with care; a chronic pain patient is as likely as anyone else to suffer acute pain that requires attention. But when there is no reason to believe that the pain is anything other than that which has been around for months or years, then take no notice of it. Do not offer pain-relieving drugs (these would reward pain behavior) or try in any way to ease the sufferer's pain. Instead, support the sufferer and respond very positively when he or she acts in a way that denies any pain; encourage "well" behavior—any activity that is normal for a well person but which may have become rare or have been dropped altogether by the pain patient.

When the patient gets up and goes out shopping or walking the dog for the first time for months it should be a cause for celebration. Every step forward should be rewarded, and steps back quietly ignored. Carers should not chide the patient for backsliding, showing pain or asking for attention; they should carry on as though nothing were happening. Punishments (even the most subtle social punishments) have unpredictable deleterious effects.

(e) Pain-control exercises

There are mental exercises that can be learned by anyone who suffers from pain problems. A technique called "cognitive pain management" has been found to be very effective for pain control. It takes some weeks to learn, but if you persevere the benefits can be enormous. If you can enlist the help of a psychologist who knows about this technique you may find it easier, though if you do not have access to such help you can work on it by yourself.

Cognitive pain management relies on the fact that pain control is a skill which can be learned. Effectively, you train yourself to interpret painful sensations in a new way. As with learning any other new skill, you will need to practice for a long time before you can control your pain; and it must be acknowledged that while some people benefit very considerably from practicing cognitive pain management, others gain little. But you have nothing to lose by trying it— and you could be one of the lucky ones! Most people get at least some relief from pain when they learn this method.

The first phase involves practicing pain control on a part of the body (ideally your right hand) that is not a pain problem for you. You learn to control sensation in a nonpainful area and then transfer that learning to painful parts.

Sit or lie in a relaxed fashion, without distractions, and close your eyes. Imagine that your hand has no sensation at all. It is made of rubber, with no feeling whatever. Look at it with your mind's eye; it might as well be dead; it looks and feels like rubber.

Practice imagining that your hand has no feeling for fifteen minutes in the morning and fifteen minutes in the evening. Teach yourself this total block of sensation so thoroughly that you can switch it on and imagine complete inability to feel pain in your hand every time you decide to do so. When you can do this, practice it every day for a week so that that knowledge is unshakably in your mind.

When you have achieved this, go on to the next phase. Place your rubber hand on a part of your body that hurts. Just leave it there, and practice imagining that it is incapable of feeling anything. You will find that it is much more difficult to do this when your hand is lying on a painful part, but if you have got the first stage right you should be able to do it after a while. Practice this second stage for fifteen minutes every morning and evening for a week.

When you can imagine total lack of sensation in the hand that lies on the painful part you will be ready for the final stage. What you do is transfer your learning from the nonpainful part to the part that hurts. You may find that it helps to leave the rubber hand on the painful part while you imagine insensitivity spreading out from it. If you practice regularly, at least twice a day, you should be capable of imagining that the previously painful part feels like rubber too. You can then cut off your perception of pain at will.

This type of mental control has long been used in Asia; the fakir on his bed of nails is a familiar cartoon character, but he does exist in reality. It is necessary to believe that you can control your pain perception, to relax and discard fear of pain (at least for a while). Tell yourself you can do it, practice, and practice again. It is not quick but it is possible. Once you have mastered this technique, you can apply it to any pain you feel, anywhere in your body.

(f) Nerve stimulation

Minute electric shocks into the skin can very effectively block some types of pain—particularly neuralgia, shingles pain and other pains caused by nerve damage. You will need a special piece of equipment called a transcutaneous nerve stimulator, which your doctor will be able to obtain for you.

12.12   BACK PAIN

While the techniques for pain control described above are appropriate to pain from any cause, back pain sufferers can benefit from specific action designed to deal with their particular problem. Four out of five people have severe backache at some time in their lives and almost everybody gets the occasional twinge—yet 90% of all backache is avoidable. It is usually caused by mechanical strains and stresses to which we become more vulnerable with age. Degenerative changes in the spine can occur through disease and are especially common among cigarette smokers, whose blood is short of oxygen which is essential to maintain the health of the discs in the spinal column. Faulty behavior patterns such as poor posture and poor lifting techniques are common causes. The precise cause of back pain is often unknown and there may be no apparent abnormality. Usually there is no underlying serious disease.

The secret of avoiding backache is to think about your back during all your everyday activities; don't wait until your back forces itself into your awareness. The most important part of your strategy for reducing back problems should be to reduce the strain involved in everyday actions. Bad posture when sitting or standing is a very common problem; muscles which have become weak through underuse increase susceptibility. Your back can be expected to give you trouble if you are not habitually active, if you do not do exercises that will strengthen your back, and if you tend to slouch. When you lift something that is too heavy, or stoop for too long, you will strain your back.

(a) Posture

Avoid letting yourself fall into a slouched, slumped posture, whether you are standing or sitting, but do not go to the other extreme and stand at attention; that puts a strain on the back too. Make sure you sit and stand tall, as though suspended from a cord from the ceiling. Try not to slip sideways; when you are standing, distribute your weight evenly on both your feet. If you have to stand for a long time, put one foot on a stool and change feet every few minutes. This reduces strain on lower back muscles.

Sitting is more hazardous to the back than standing, largely because we have adopted a style of furniture which is not best designed to suit our backs. If you sit for a long time each day, make sure you have a chair that gives good support to the lower part of the spine. If necessary adapt your chair to meet your needs with a small cushion or a length of fabric wound around the back of the chair and padded to match the shape of your back, or a backrest made specifically for the purpose. Avoid beanbag chairs, chairs that you sink into and chairs with seats longer than your thighs which force you into a slouched position.

Driving in a heavily worn or badly designed seat can readily induce backache, especially if driving makes you tense. Make sure you are always sitting up very straight when driving, and consciously relax your shoulders. If you drive a lot you may need a special backrest. Some chronic backache victims have cured their problem by getting new seats fitted to their cars.

Never sit for more than an hour without getting up. Whether you are driving, doing office work or writing, you should stop every hour to stretch your legs. Your work will improve and your back will benefit.

Sleeping in a soft bed can also be hazardous to the back. Choose a firm mattress or put a plywood board between the bed base and the mattress. If you sleep on your back, place a pillow or cushion under your knees so that they are slightly bent. If you are more comfortable on your side, use a pillow that keeps your head properly aligned with your spine and bend your knees. Don't sleep on your stomach, don't sleep on a waterbed and don't read in bed.

(b) Lifting and carrying

Most people have weak backs because they have not devoted enough time to strengthening their back muscles. When people with weak back muscles try to lift heavy weights they risk injury. Strengthen your back with the exercise routines referred to in section 17.6. Avoid carrying weights whenever you can; using a cart or dolly is always better than carrying a load. Get a shopping cart or use a bicycle for shopping if you carry your groceries home.

When you do have to lift or carry weights, try to let your legs do as much of the work as possible. Keep the weight close to your body and lift no higher than the waist. Never turn at the waist; turn instead from the feet. Avoid carrying a weight on only one side of your body; carry two suitcases rather than one. Don't try to carry too much at a time. If you are shoveling, keep the quantities on your spade or shovel small. Divide the contents of a box of groceries into smaller packages for transfer from grocery cart to car. Kneel when appropriate to lift heavy items from floor level. Squat like a weight lifter to bring your shoulders to the level of the thing you have to lift. Avoid stooping or bending for long periods; if you like gardening, use long-handled tools which reduce the need for stooping wherever possible. Kneel on a mat instead of bending when you are weeding or planting.

If you are in any doubt about suitable postures for reducing strain on the back, borrow a book on the subject from your local library.

(c) Exercises

Stretching exercises can help ease a painful back; strengthening exercises will reduce your future back problems. Whenever you do exercises for your back, it is important that you do not jerk or force your body into any desired position. Keep as relaxed as you can and move quite slowly and smoothly.

Stretch your neck by bending the head forward, backward and to each side. Then turn your head as far as possible each way so that you are looking behind you. Don't blend the movements together into a circling motion; keep them separate and repeat the sequence.

Stretch your whole back by hanging on a bar or climbing frame; if you have no special equipment just put on a pair of thick gloves and hang by your hands from a sturdy door. Choose a spot near the hinges so you don't pull it out of its frame. Relax your legs so that the weight of your body stretches your spine and swing gently from side to side. Put the weight back on your legs carefully. If you are able to hang upside down by the knees from a climbing frame, the weight of your head will stretch your neck. Do not, however, attempt to do pull-ups or tense your arms or back; this will interfere with the stretching.

Jogging and running can add to back problems because of the pounding which may be transmitted through the spine. If you want the aerobic benefit of this type of activity, make sure you have bouncy running shoes, run on grass whenever possible and run on your toes rather than landing hard on your heels. An indoor minitrampoline will facilitate enjoyable jumping and running on the spot without jarring your back.

Swimming is the ideal form of exercise for back sufferers. Go as often as you can and swim as long as you like. The more you do, the more your whole body will benefit.

(d) Hints for soothing back pain

If your back is very sore you will want to lie down. Warmth is helpful; a heated pad is ideal, but a hot-water bottle or electric blanket on the back will do (but don't have it so warm that you burn your skin!). While you are lying down, take the opportunity to reach as far as you can with your toes, stretching first one foot then the other.

After injury to the back, normal strength takes at least six weeks to return; a second injury will take longer to recover from. So if you have had one episode of severe back pain, make sure you take precautions to avoid another. Build up strength gradually but surely with exercise.

Most minor back pains do not require bed rest, and sufferers generally do not recover any faster if they stay in bed for longer than acute pain necessitates. However, if your back problem came at a time of general overstrain, bed rest might be exactly what you need. After that, gentle movement will help speed repair, but take care not to strain your back again.

(e) Back care products

You can buy furniture that is designed with the back in mind. Special seats which minimize back strain are available from back care stores. You can even get made-to-measure chairs—if you can afford them!

For those who do a lot of reading, a lectern that clips to your desk can reduce neck strain, while a tilting, adjustable desk may be helpful if your back pain is related to the strain of working on a horizontal surface. Vibrating or heating cushions can relieve back pain, but you should not use a vibrating cushion for more than ten minutes in any hour.

13

Arthritis, Rheumatism and Joint Problems

This chapter covers aches and pains in the joints and associated structures, including all types of arthritis and rheumatism, gout, bursitis, sprains and stiffness due to injury or other causes.

Joint problems are very common, but they rarely cause serious problems for young people. Osteoarthritis is the most common form of joint disorder; it is often seen as the inevitable result of aging, a result of a lifetime's wear and tear. However, the pain, stiffness, disability and potential deformity produced by joint problems are very much dependent on the way we treat ourselves.

Rheumatism is the general term for all sorts of joint disorders. It includes both arthritis and muscle or joint pain from other causes such as strains and virus infections. Often it will clear up of its own accord.

Bursitis is the term used for an inflammation of the connective tissues of a joint. It is a very common industrial injury. It normally clears up by itself but is liable to recur.

SECTION INDEX

13.1 *Strains, sprains and bursitis*
13.2 *Gout*
13.3 *Drugs for gout*
13.4 *Alternatives to drugs for gout*
13.5 *Arthritis and rheumatism*
13.6 *Drugs for arthritis*
13.7 *Alternatives to drugs for arthritis*
13.8 *Organizations for arthritis sufferers*

13.1 STRAINS, SPRAINS AND BURSITIS

These conditions are all results of injury to the muscles, ligaments and other tissues that surround, support and move a joint.

Bursitis is a frequent result of overuse of a joint such as the wrist; it is an inflammation of the sheath that covers the ligaments and tendons. Soreness and weakness develop when a particular joint has been used too much—for example, in the wrist after a day's bricklaying or vigorous tennis at the beginning of the season. Housemaid's knee, tennis elbow, dustman's shoulder, miner's elbow and weaver's bottom are all forms of bursitis.

Strains and sprains are caused by sudden excessive demands on the joint which can bruise and stretch or tear the ligaments. Soothe the pain with cold compresses (bags of frozen peas are excellent) and reduce swelling by keeping the affected part raised, ideally above waist level.

Recovery from all these conditions requires rest, so try to use the joint as little as possible until the discomfort has gone. Knee injuries (such as often afflict skiers) may take two months to heal. An elastic bandage or sling which supports the joint will help. No other action is required.

13.2   GOUT

Gout causes a sudden and severe pain in a joint, most often the big toe. It is the result of an accumulation of uric acid in the tissues, and the cause is likely to be the metabolic imbalance induced by drugs such as diuretics. If you get an attack of gout, do *not* take aspirin; it will make matters worse.

13.3   DRUGS FOR GOUT

Acute attacks of gout are treated with antiinflammatory analgesic drugs such as those listed in section 12.10(*b*). Indomethacin (Indocin) is usually used. Drugs for long-term control of gout are allopurinol (Lopurin, Zyloprim), probenecid (Benemid, Col-Probenecid) and sulfinpyrazone (Anturane).

Allopurinol reduces the formation of uric acid, while probenecid and sulfinpyrazone increase the excretion of uric acid. Neither allopurinol nor probenecid should be taken during or shortly after an acute attack of gout; they can make the problem worse. Side effects of these drugs include rashes, nausea, gastrointestinal problems, malaise, headache, dizziness, hair loss, liver and kidney damage and blood disorders. If you take any of these drugs, increase the amount of water you drink to help prevent the formation of crystals in the urine.

13.4   ALTERNATIVES TO DRUGS FOR GOUT

If you are taking drugs that may affect your metabolism, especially diuretics (usually prescribed for high blood pressure and other circulatory problems), study section 9.11 on alternatives to drugs for heart disease. It should be possible to reduce the dose you take and gradually eliminate your need for these drugs. Your gout problem is then likely to disappear.

If you are not taking any drugs on a regular basis, then you should change your diet. Gout is associated with a level of alcohol consumption which is too high for your body, and with diets rich in animal products. Our forefathers were quite right to blame pheasant and port wine! Eat less meat and dairy produce, increase your intake of vegetables and grains, and try to substitute pure mineral water for alcoholic drinks as often as possible; in other words, eat and drink as we recommend in section 18.2. This will cause the level of uric acid in your body to fall and you should cease to suffer from gout.

13.5   ARTHRITIS AND RHEUMATISM

Joint pains that begin unexpectedly are usually symptoms of infection, and they normally disappear quite quickly. Take things easy, and make sure you are getting enough sleep and a diet rich in vitamin C (section 18.4(f)). Warmth is likely to be helpful.

Long-lasting joint pain, which may come on slowly or start with an illness somewhat akin to a virus infection that goes on and on, is due to arthritis. Arthritis is thought to be a collection of disorders with a range of causes. Although no remedy can be expected to cure most arthritis completely, almost every sufferer can reduce the effects of arthritic joints by self-management techniques (see section 13.7). The same technique will not offer the same benefit for all sufferers; your own experience is the best guide to which approach is best for you. But do try to give each method an unprejudiced trial. Give it at least two weeks, preferably a month, before deciding whether it is helpful; shorter trials are not likely to be reliable. Remember, arthritic joints take years to get damaged, so you cannot expect any fast results. In fact, quick results are potentially dangerous, whether they come from drugs or any other form of treatment; the symptoms may just be masked while the damage to your joints gets worse. You will have to be patient and adjust your thinking to the same slow time scale as the disease. But be reassured; arthritis becomes less severe with time as the condition stabilizes.

13.6   DRUGS FOR ARTHRITIS

The drugs most often prescribed for arthritis and similar conditions are aspirin and related products—the nonsteroidal anti-inflammatory analgesics (NSAIs) listed in section 12.10. These tend to reduce the swelling and inflammation in affected joints as well as reducing the pain. They do not affect the disease process; they merely suppress the symptoms somewhat.

Sufferers from severe arthritis may be given a range of other drugs when treatment with NSAIs has proved insufficient to slow the progress of the disease. Gold, in the form of aurothioglucose (Solganal) or gold sodium thiomalate (Myochrysine) injections, and penicillamine (Cuprimine, Depen) do not produce their full benefits for some months, and adverse reactions can be fatal. Severe reactions to gold injections occur in one in twenty patients. Side effects of both drugs include mouth ulcers, skin reactions, water retention and blood disease (sometimes sudden and fatal). Gold occasionally causes colitis, nerve damage and lung problems; penicillamine can also cause hypersensitivity reactions, nausea, taste loss, muscle weakness, fever and systemic lupus erythematosus (a disease with many features similar to severe rheumatoid arthritis).

Chloroquine (Aralen) is an antimalarial drug which is sometimes used for arthritis. Adverse effects include irreversible damage to the eyes, skin reactions, gastrointestinal problems, headache, hair loss, hearing problems and blood disorders.

Rheumatic disease can also be treated with steroids, synthetic forms of natural hormones which reduce inflammation (see section 6.4(d)). Hailed as wonder drugs when they were discovered to be capable of giving immediate relief to arthritis sufferers, steroids have fallen into disfavor because of their serious adverse effects. They are still prescribed occasionally for people with severe disease that does not respond to other measures, but they should not be used until all alternative strategies have been exhausted. Steroids can be injected directly into affected joints. This may give immediate relief but the effects do not usually last. Repeated injections into a joint can cause permanent damage and make the area vulnerable to infection. Uncontrollable infections that start under these circumstances can kill.

13.7   ALTERNATIVES TO DRUGS FOR ARTHRITIS

One important fact about all these conditions is that they are much more common in Western industrial countries than in poorer countries. Although arthritis exists all over the world, and has been known for thousands of years, it is made worse by our way of life. This strongly suggests that the cause of at least some forms of arthritis lies in our life-style, and therefore that the best way to deal with it must be making life-style changes.

(a) Diet

For some sufferers, joint inflammation is a symptom of allergy. These people can achieve dramatic benefits by identifying and avoiding those substances (usually foods) to which they are allergic. Accumulating clinical evidence now supports the experience of sufferers that arthritis and other joint problems can be ameliorated and sometimes even cured by the adoption of a special diet.

Patricia Byrivers, author of *Goodbye to Arthritis,* discovered that the severe form of rheumatoid arthritis from which she had suffered since her teens was allergic in origin. By avoiding particular foods she has been able to achieve and maintain spectacular improvements in this supposedly incurable condition, and she explains how other sufferers can work out whether their illness is related to food or chemical allergy.

Anecdotal evidence from arthritics attributes improvement to avoidance of a wide range of foods. Dairy products (cow's milk, cream, cheese and any prepared foods containing milk products) are particularly often held responsible for flare-ups of joint pain. (See section 18.8.) As with all problems of food allergy, it is important that you do not go overboard in eliminating foods and end up inadequately nourished. Recovery requires good nutrition. But you will not come to any harm if you cut out one group of foods at a time, replacing it with other sources of the same nutrients. For example, you might avoid all cow's-milk products for two weeks, and use soya milk instead; or give up all wheat and flour-based products for a similar period, substituting rice and potatoes for bread, cakes, cookies, and pasta.

If you do not want to go through the rigors of an elimination diet, you could try changing to a Japanese-style diet high in organic brown rice, vegetables and fish; this automatically removes the most common food allergens. However, you cannot expect to find out if it works

for you unless you eat this way consistently and at every meal. You will
need a suitable cookbook for guidance; one which has been shown to
help arthritics is *Dr. Dong's Arthritis Cookbook*. The foods which Dr.
Dong suggests arthritics should avoid include dairy produce, red meat,
citrus fruits, vinegar, alcohol and anything containing certain additives such as monosodium glutamate (MSG). While this diet does not
help everyone, it produces excellent benefits for some.

Mineral balance may also be important in rheumatic disease and
arthritis. The traditional use of a copper bracelet has been vindicated
by research which demonstrated low copper levels in the blood in
many sufferers. Try it; it is too easy a step to neglect. It will make your
skin turn green at the point of contact but you should not worry
about that; the copper salts that you absorb through your skin just
happen to be green.

It has been suggested that excessive iron adds to our problems.
Whether it does so directly or indirectly by interfering with use of
other minerals is not clear, but the implication for arthritis sufferers is
that they should avoid taking iron supplements.

(b) Activity and exercises to ease joint problems

It is essential that arthritic joints be used in order to maintain
mobility and avoid disablement. But it is equally important that you
do not overuse diseased joints, because this will delay healing. Rest
reduces inflammation, which is good, but it also leads to stiffness and
muscle wastage.

Exercises should be done regularly, frequently and with care. The
general principle is that you should take each joint through its full
range of movement every day, coaxing it gently a fraction further
than it wants to go, just past the point of discomfort, and then relax.
Research has confirmed that people who exercise at least three days
every week, or practice relaxation or other techniques specifically
designed to reduce their arthritis problems, have significantly less
pain, are more active and need to consult their doctors less often
than those who do not. It does not matter how severe your disease is;
you can always improve your condition.

Exercise your joints when the pain and stiffness are at their minimum level and when you are not feeling tired. For most people this happens at much the same time every day, so make this the regular time for your mobility exercises. Don't choose a time when your pain has been reduced with drugs, and *never* take tablets to reduce the inflammation so that you can do more exercises. Use your pain as a guide to the amount you can do; if you override it too much, you risk damaging your joints further.

Always warm up before exercise. Start your day by stretching all over before you get out of bed; imagine you are a cat and stretch all your limbs and your back. Take up one of the general body-conditioning exercises that are of particular benefit to arthritis sufferers—swimming, cycling or walking. Ideally you should do ten to fifteen minutes of exercise every day. Swimming is the most effective form of activity for people with joint problems; telephone your local pools to find out if there is a time set aside for therapeutic use. Check also on the temperature of the pools; you will want to use the warmest one. Pools that are used by young children are often better heated than large adult pools. Private health clubs sometimes also have well-heated swimming or exercise pools.

Cycling is particularly good for maintaining mobility in the hips and knees. Build up gently, make sure your bike is well maintained and lubricated so that pedal action is not stiff, and keep in low gear so that you use minimum force. Aim to build up speed in first gear and don't shift upward even if it seems effortless; try to move your legs faster. A static exercise bike can be good, but again you must be sure to keep the pedal resistance low so that you move your legs as fast as possible.

Walking, too, is valuable; equip yourself with a pair of comfortable running shoes (from a specialized sports store) and try to get out on foot every day. If you have arthritic hips, legs or ankles you may have to get your weight down through careful eating and regular swimming or cycling before you can benefit from walking.

(c) *Exercises to mobilize damaged joints*

You should begin your exercise routine with small movements that don't cause pain. These can be derived from exercises such as those described below, or just a good shake. Heat painful and stiff joints prior to exercise; a hot bath or shower is good, or use an electric heating pad, a hot-water bottle or any suitable heater. If a joint is hot because of arthritis, just move that joint through its full range of movements twice daily. Exercise with a slow, steady rhythm, breathing deeply throughout. Never stress arthritic joints with weights or pressure.

Arthritis most often affects the hands. You can reduce the disablement and strengthen them by doing regular hand exercises. If your hands are particularly stiff you may find it helpful to do your exercises in a basin of warm water. One method which is good for arthritic knuckles and fingers is to bend the fingers slowly, one at a time, toward the palm. Then push each one a little further with the other hand. Try making an O between your thumb and each finger in turn, pressing the tips together for a few seconds. Practice also putting your palm flat on a table and straightening your fingers, pushing down carefully as you do so.

Arthritic shoulders can be helped by bending over at the waist, hanging your arms in front of your body and making horizontal circles of increasing size with your hands. Try another exercise: hold a cane or broom handle with your hands a yard apart and raise it as high overhead as you can. Or take a rope or dressing-gown cord and throw it over an open door, holding one end in each hand; pull down on one end so that your other arm is raised up; coax the arm a little higher than it wants to go and then pull down with it, raising the first arm.

To exercise an arthritic neck, drop your chin to your chest and let your head fall as far forward as it will go. Then slowly drop your head backward. Tilt your head to the left and to the right. Turn to look over each shoulder in turn.

If your arthritis affects your hips, choose movements which are particularly limited and concentrate on them, stretching just past the point of discomfort. One exercise to improve sideways mobility is done lying on the back with your legs raised vertically, your feet in the air. Keeping your legs straight, spread them as far apart as possible, then coax them a little further using your hands. Or lying on your back with legs vertical, keep one leg straight and pull the other knee down toward your chest with your hand under your thigh. Straighten and repeat with the other leg. Repeat these movements as often as you like, but avoid more than minor discomfort. Turn onto your front for a strengthening exercise: raise each leg in turn, as high as possible.

Arthritic knees should be exercised without putting weight on them. Lie on your back with both knees bent and bring one knee toward your chest. Using your hands to assist, gently bend the knee as far as you can; then do the same for the other knee. Try also bending each knee as far as possible when sitting on a firm chair; then sit on the floor with your legs out in front of you to practice straightening the knees.

Arthritic ankles should be stretched and bent alternately to their maximum extent. Try sitting on a chair with your feet flat on the floor. Raise your toes as high as you can with your heels still on the ground. Then, with your toes on the ground, raise your heels as high as possible. Repeat, moving your feet to one side and then the other, raising toes and heels alternately in a dance.

Use your imagination to design your exercise regime to meet your special needs. Begin slowly and aim for mobility in every direction in which a normal joint will move. Then work on each diseased joint gently. It is often a good idea to use passive movement, using your hands to pull the limb or body part you are working on just a little further than it would otherwise be able to go. But always take care not to cause yourself anything more than slight discomfort, and discontinue anything that makes your joint hurt more than two hours after the exercise session. When this happens it means you are pushing it too far. Take it easy; patience will be rewarded with steady improvement.

(d) Protecting damaged joints

While stretching and mobilizing exercises will help you to regain full use of your joints, you should be careful not to overload them and damage them further through everyday activity. Try to avoid ordinary actions that give you pain. Use special devices to adapt appliances to meet your needs whenever possible. A wide range of these devices is available; doorknob extenders, button hooks for clothes, and special can openers are just some of them. Contact any of the arthritis support groups listed in section 13.8 for advice and information.

Make full use of other devices that are not designed specifically for arthritics but which can help, such as wheeled luggage-carriers, old-fashioned clothespins instead of spring-loaded ones, vegetable choppers and food processors. Use your imagination to work out ways of overcoming difficulties—for example, by tying a strap to cupboard or refrigerator handles so that you can use your arm rather than your hand to open them. Push drawers shut with your hip rather than stressing arthritic hands or wrists, and use both hands where most people would use one—for example, to hold cups and plates. Have unnecessary doors removed from cupboards and eliminate unnecessary tasks from your life. Perhaps you should relax your standards of housekeeping or acknowledge that your garden won't be as perfect as it once was.

Finally, ask others to help when something puts a strain on your joints. They won't know what causes difficulties for you and most people are only too glad to assist. Don't be embarrassed; there really is no need to be self-conscious about arthritis!

13.8   ORGANIZATIONS FOR ARTHRITIS SUFFERERS

Arthritis Foundation, 1314 Spring St. NW, Atlanta, GA 30309. (404) 872–7100.

Information Center for Individuals with Disabilities, 20 Park Plz., Room 330, Boston, MA 02116. (617) 727–5540.

Accent on Information, P.O. Box 700, Bloomington, IL 61702. (309) 378–2961. Computerized information on aids and services for people with disabilities.

14

The Reproductive System

This chapter deals with a wide range of genital and reproductive problems. They include vaginal and vulval itching and soreness; thrush, herpes and other infections; problems associated with the menstrual cycle such as menstrual pain, heavy periods, loss of periods and premenstrual syndrome; contraception, infertility and impotence; and ailments affecting the penis.

Women frequently experience problems with their reproductive systems. For many they are the only reasons for consulting their doctor; indeed, it is because of these "female" ailments that women consult their doctor considerably more often than men. Genital infections are also very common. They rarely clear up spontaneously.

SECTION INDEX

14.1   *The female reproductive system*
14.2   *Premenstrual syndrome (PMS)*
14.3   *Drugs for PMS*

225

14.4　*Alternatives to drugs for PMS*
14.5　*Menstrual pain*
14.6　*Drugs for menstrual pain*
14.7　*Alternatives to drugs for menstrual pain*
14.8　*Missed periods*
14.9　*Heavy periods*
14.10　*Contraceptive drugs*
14.11　*Alternatives to drugs for contraception*
14.12　*Infertility*
14.13　*Drugs for infertility*
14.14　*Alternatives to drugs for infertility*
14.15　*Vaginal and vulval itching and soreness (vaginitis)*
14.16　*Vaginal thrush (candidiasis)*
14.17　*Drugs for thrush*
14.18　*Alternatives to drugs for thrush*
14.19　*Other vaginal infections*
14.20　*Herpes*
14.21　*Drugs for herpes*
14.22　*Alternatives to drugs for herpes*
14.23　*Infections of the penis*
14.24　*Impotence*

14.1　THE FEMALE REPRODUCTIVE SYSTEM

The constant cycling of the woman's sex hormones affects the state of her reproductive system—and indeed her whole body—throughout her fertile years. From the beginning of menstruation until menopause, women move constantly through a repeating monthly cycle, its pattern broken only by pregnancy, severe stress or ill health, or medical intervention. It is a powerful cycle that affects their moods, their sense of well-being, their interests and their susceptibility to illness; and it is in turn affected by their activities and way of life.

The cycle and its effects vary tremendously from woman to woman. Broadly speaking, all women from the age of about twelve to fifty bleed at intervals of around twenty-eight days; the bleeding continues for a few days. Twelve to fourteen days after the beginning of each period, the levels of three major sex hormones—estrogen, luteinizing hormone and follicle-stimulating hormone—peak and fall with ovulation (the production of a microscopic egg). At this time there may be abdominal pain (usually short-lived and quite slight), an upsurge of sexual interest, a certain unpredictability and enhanced intensity of emotion. After ovulation the levels of another hormone, progesterone, rise; then in the last week or so of the month, as progesterone falls again, many women feel tense and heavy. Bleeding begins when all these hormones are at a low level.

The onset of menstrual bleeding varies tremendously in its significance for different women. It can be a blessed relief from premenstrual tension or something to be dreaded because of the pain that regularly accompanies it; both patterns are common and some women experience both. It may also be welcomed or resented as evidence of nonpregnancy. Many doctors (predominantly male) believe that menstruation is important to women as confirmation of their femininity, which is one reason why oral contraceptives are given for three weeks out of four, producing a fall in hormone levels and monthly "withdrawal bleeding."

The vagina, vulva (the area around the entrance to the vagina) and reproductive organs are delicate parts of women's bodies. The membranes are sensitive and vulnerable to infection, and the balance of the hormones is readily upset, producing a wide range of problems affecting all systems of the body. Indeed, for many women in their childbearing years, such specifically female problems are the most important cause of illness, both major and minor.

Because of the embarrassment that many people feel when discussing sexual matters there is widespread ignorance about the reproductive organs. There can be great uncertainty, for example, about what is normal and what is not, and there are times when commercial interests play on our fears, making matters much worse than they need be. Anatomical variations between women are quite wide. In some the inner lips of the vagina extend beyond the outer; this is perfectly normal.

Some discharge from the vagina is also normal; it carries your unique smell which is designed to be naturally attractive to men, and it lubricates the vagina so that you do not get sore. Most women produce more discharge in the middle of the month, around ovulation; at this time it tends to change slightly in consistency. It is sensible to get to know the smell and qualities of your healthy discharge because then you will be able to tell when something is going wrong; the smell, quantity and other characteristics of the discharge will change if you have an infection.

14.2 PREMENSTRUAL SYNDROME (PMS)

Premenstrual syndrome (PMS) is a very common condition in women from fourteen to fifty. It starts three to ten days before the beginning of the menstrual period and continues sometimes until the second day of the period. Symptoms are of two types, mental and physical. No single symptom is definitive; different women show different patterns. The most common symptoms are mood fluctuations, ranging from extreme excitability, irritability and aggression to black depression and weepiness. Many women lose confidence, concentration and coordination, becoming absentminded and inefficient. Of the physical problems the most common are caused by fluid retention: abdominal bloating, swelling of hands, feet, legs and face—sometimes the whole body. The breasts may swell and become sore through hormone changes. Persistent tiredness, headache, backache and skin problems similar to acne are not uncommon. There may be a marked loss of interest in sex. Symptoms of long-standing illness may become more severe.

Other symptoms of PMS include pain similar to menstrual pain, spontaneous bruising especially of the legs, irritation of the lining of the nose and eyes, blotchy spots on the face and neck, joint pains, constipation, vertigo, migraine, bingeing on food or alcohol and craving for foods such as chocolate.

Many of these symptoms are familiar to most women, and they may occur independently of hormone changes. The only way you can tell is by keeping a diary of your emotional and health problems and looking for any relationship between your symptoms and the timing of your menstrual cycle. Often the link is very obvious. If, for example, a nameless dread overwhelms you with miserable regularity four days before each period, then you are likely to benefit considerably from measures designed to alleviate PMS.

14.3 DRUGS FOR PMS

Some doctors will prescribe a whole variety of drugs to suppress premenstrual symptoms. If you get overwrought, they may offer tranquilizers; if you have pain, they'll suggest analgesics; if you're bloated, you'll get diuretics. Obviously these remedies do not get to the root of the problem, and since the premenstrual syndrome has many unpleasant facets, you're likely to continue to suffer until you can deal with the cause of your hormone imbalance.

Doctors who attribute PMS to lack of progesterone in the second half of the menstrual cycle may prescribe progesterone. Natural progesterone works well for 30% of women but has no benefit for another 30%; the remaining 40% get partial relief. Progesterone can cause weight gain but has no serious adverse effects.

14.4 ALTERNATIVES TO DRUGS FOR PMS

Just as there are tremendous variations in the precise pattern of symptoms of premenstrual syndrome, so there are equal variations in response to different types of treatment. You will have to discover your personal answer by trial and error.

(a) Nutrition

Pyridoxine (vitamin B_6) supplements help the majority of PMS sufferers even if their diet is rich in this vitamin. (It is found in whole-grain bread and other whole grain products, meat, milk, eggs and yeast; see section 18.4(e) for other sources.) Begin by taking a 50 mg. tablet or capsule, morning and evening, from three days before you anticipate the onset of PMS symptoms until the beginning of your period. If this does not relieve your symptoms effectively, try raising the dose to 150 mg. daily, but do not exceed this dose because you may suffer from an unpleasant acid stomach. Once you are free from PMS symptoms, try cutting the dose back down to 50 mg. daily; this is often sufficient. Pyridoxine is particularly effective for the relief of mood changes, breast discomfort and headaches.

Gamma-linoleic acid (GLA) in the form of evening primrose oil or blackcurrant seed oil is another valuable nutritional supplement for PMS sufferers. Various brands are available from health-food stores and pharmacists; use it in much the same way as pyridoxine, experimenting with the dose until you find the level at which your symptoms disappear. Many PMS sufferers find that they no longer require GLA after a few months of use, especially if they eat a diet rich in unprocessed oils and trace minerals. Nuts and seeds, avocados, fresh fish and cold-pressed olive, sunflower and other oils are particularly valuable.

All PMS sufferers should ensure that they eat enough food during the second half of the cycle. Don't skip meals and don't try to cut calories. Eat plenty of fresh fruit, especially citrus fruit, and vegetables. PMS sufferers tend to have lower-than-average magnesium levels; check section 18.4(l) for foods rich in magnesium and incorporate more of these into your diet. However, modern farming and food processing mean that your diet could be deficient in magnesium even if you take care to eat well. Supplements of chelated magnesium may be helpful.

During your premenstrual days you may be more sensitive to the effects of drugs, including those in everyday drinks. You may get drunk more easily on alcohol and develop a headache more readily afterward, and you may get more irritable on coffee and cola (see section 18.9). Think twice before taking any drugs when you are premenstrual.

If you suffer from bloating, try solidago (goldenrod) tea, which is a natural diuretic.

(b) Exercise

Quite strenuous exercise can be helpful in combating PMS. It relieves mental and physical tension and promotes efficient functioning throughout the body. It relieves depression and aids sound sleep. However, you may find it very difficult to motivate yourself to start any activity, and poor coordination may mean that your performance is worse than at other times of the month.

Don't expect too much of yourself, but try not to let yourself slump either. Read chapter 17, especially sections 17.2, 17.4, 17.6, 17.7 and 17.9, for some suggestions.

14.5 MENSTRUAL PAIN

Menstrual pain, like PMS, takes a variety of forms. Some women, especially those under twenty-five, suffer from spasms of colicky pain in the lower abdomen, particularly during the first day of the period. After pregnancy this type of pain often disappears. A heavy, continuous type of pain in the lower abdomen is more common among mature women. It may begin before the period, and can get worse after pregnancy. Many women who also suffer from PMS get this sort of pain; when this is the case, treating the PMS will often prevent the onset of menstrual pain.

Some doctors used to believe that menstrual pain was a sign of emotional problems. There is no evidence to support this, though the association between PMS and pain might have contributed to the development of the idea. The idea that it is a neurotic symptom may still color the attitudes of some doctors, and the fact that most doctors are male and have no experience of the problem, coupled with the fact that it is not life-threatening, means that many do not take it seriously.

Medical help is usually not necessary for menstrual problems. However, if the pain is very much more severe than you have come to expect, it could be a symptom of pelvic infection. Consult a doctor without delay if your pain is definitely much worse than in previous months, if you have had an IUD for three months or more, or if you have had intercourse with a new lover or a man you share with another woman. Pelvic pain accompanied by nausea and fever is likely to require urgent medical treatment.

14.6 DRUGS FOR MENSTRUAL PAIN

The drugs normally used for menstrual pain are over-the-counter analgesics (see section 5.3), though antispasmodic drugs such as scopolamine (Donnagel, Donnatal) (section 8.6(*a*)) are also said to help. Choose aspirin or ibuprofen rather than acetaminophen for menstrual pain; you will find them more effective because they have antiprostaglandin properties. None of these drugs are likely to produce any adverse effects when taken occasionally in low doses, unless you are particularly sensitive to them. If you need a stronger painkiller, ask your doctor for an anti-inflammatory drug such as naproxen (section 12.10).

If you decide to take an analgesic, choose one that has antiprostaglandin properties because this will be far more effective for menstrual pain than one which does not.

Sex hormones may be prescribed for menstrual pain; many girls have been put on the Pill for this reason, ostensibly at least.

14.7   ALTERNATIVES TO DRUGS FOR MENSTRUAL PAIN

Many of the actions you can take to relieve PMS will also help with menstrual pain by rebalancing your hormone systems. It should not be necessary, and it is certainly not desirable, to take doses of hormones in tablet form when you can get your own body to produce the right levels for you. Study section 14.4 on alternatives to drugs for PMS. GLA (evening primrose oil) may be particularly valuable in preventing menstrual pain.

Exercise before your period will often reduce problems when the bleeding starts. Consistently high exercise levels throughout the month can reduce bleeding to the point where periods cease altogether, though you will experience improvements well before this! Cycling and swimming in the days preceding the expected onset of your period will be helpful, and if you can continue to exercise when your period starts it may relieve the pain dramatically if not make it disappear completely. However, walking and running sometimes make the pain worse because they jolt the pelvic organs.

When menstrual pain is at its worst you may feel far too tired to start exercising. Try a very hot bath; just lie there, reheating the bath with hot water as often as necessary till the pain has faded. Then go to bed with a hot-water bottle.

Constipation makes menstrual pain worse. See section 18.3 for a diet that will prevent it.

Many women who were previously free of pain begin to experience it after the insertion of an IUD. Removal of the device will usually be sufficient to return you to your original state, though this does not always seem to happen. If you develop an infection through the use of an IUD you may find it difficult to reestablish the pain-free periods you used to have. And while you may have been told that you will have painful periods only for the first month or two, this is not the experience of many women. Judge your body's reactions carefully; pain may mean that all is not well. The convenience of this form of contraception can be outweighed by its health hazards.

14.8 MISSED PERIODS

The hormone mechanisms which control the menstrual cycle are delicately balanced and they can be thrown off by a great range of events, stresses and physiological imbalances. Because the cycle is controlled by the hormone "master gland," the pituitary, which is connected to the emotional centers of the brain, the menstrual cycle is particularly sensitive to disruption by emotional stress. Some women miss periods when important relationships break up; some will find that the period they expected during examinations never arrives; some miss periods because they are terrified they might be pregnant. Usually in such cases the gap is only one month. However, since the most common cause of missed periods is undoubtedly pregnancy, do take a pregnancy test two weeks after the expected date even if you think that stress might be the real cause.

While stress can cause some women to miss their periods, for others it can result in exceptionally heavy and painful periods. If you experience the latter, try to take time for yourself toward the end of the month; use relaxation techniques balanced with rhythmic physical activity to reduce the impact of stress hormones. Follow the advice for PMS (section 14.4) and take a higher dose of GLA in high-stress months.

Synthetic female sex hormones (estrogens) can be used to induce artificial periods in women who do not menstruate. However, since this is no more than the sort of withdrawal bleeding produced by the

Pill, and not any normalization of the menstrual cycle, the use of these potentially hazardous hormones is irrational.

If you have been menstruating regularly and then miss four or more periods in succession you should see a doctor for a thorough physical examination. The cause can be serious illness such as diabetes and may require urgent attention. Other causes (apart from pregnancy) include extreme weight loss caused by obsessive dieting, anorexia or bulimia (self-induced vomiting); excessive running or other physically demanding exercise taken to unusual extremes; extreme weight gain due to disease or compulsive eating; and severe emotional stress. In these cases, the cause is probably apparent—at least to the woman concerned—but they all (except, perhaps, competitive sport) reflect underlying psychological or social problems which demand attention because damage will be occurring in all facets of the woman's life. Even if missing periods may seem in itself a trivial symptom— perhaps a relief—the health consequences of the sort of regime that induces it will be many. The human body is not able to cope with such levels of stress for long periods without breaking down. Help from a sympathetic counselor or psychologist is probably required, but the stress-reduction methods described in chapter 16 will reduce the severity of the problem.

Sometimes periods do not return for some months after discontinuation of oral contraceptives or contraceptive injections. If this could be your problem, follow the advice for PMS in section 14.4. Your periods will probably return naturally.

14.9 HEAVY PERIODS

If your periods are becoming progressively heavier and more troublesome, you would be wise to consult a doctor. It could be a symptom of a condition such as endometriosis, fibroids or ovarian cysts for which treatment may be essential. However, if causes such as these can be eliminated, or even if a small fibroid is found, you may be able to rebalance your hormones and solve the problem. Follow the advice for PMS in section 14.4. GLA is a valuable nutritional supplement for women with these problems. You will also need to maintain your iron intake because heavy blood loss can make you anemic. See section 18.4(i) for dietary advice.

Types of activity which induce muscle-building can be helpful because they will change your body function in such a way as to counter naturally the development of menstrual problems associated with excessive estrogen production (see sections 17.7 and 17.9).

Losing fat will often help too, but don't try to do it by dieting. See section 10.8 for alternative ways.

14.10 CONTRACEPTIVE DRUGS

Oral and injected contraceptives contain synthetic forms of the female sex hormones, estrogens and progestogens. These are *not* the same as the naturally produced forms and their effects are different. They are taken daily in the form of "the Pill," or in a larger injected dose. They are designed to prevent the release of an egg (ovulation), and large doses taken after intercourse ("the morning-after pill") will prevent a fertilized egg from developing into a baby.

These drugs are highly effective if used correctly. They would undoubtedly be the preferred method of contraception for most women if it were not for their side effects. A comprehensive guide to the problems of the Pill is Dr. Ellen Grant's book *The Bitter Pill.* Dr. Grant worked for Britain's Family Planning Association and studied the Pill from its earliest days of use in Britain. At first she was enthusiastic—it seemed like the perfect contraceptive—but as the years went on she saw too much suffering, too many women with serious illness that was clearly related to the Pill. She is now totally opposed to its use.

Adverse effects of the Pill include cardiovascular disease (strokes, heart attacks, high blood pressure) and an increased risk of breast and cervical cancer. The longer you take it the more likely you are to suffer long-term damage to health. You are more likely to suffer from allergies, severe depression, migraine, diabetes and vaginal infections, and you are more likely to produce a deformed baby if you do become pregnant. The suicide rate of Pill users is significantly higher than that of women of the same age who use other contraceptive methods.

Injected forms of similar hormones (Depo-Provera) have not been in use for as long, or in so many women, so their adverse effects are not as well documented. Nevertheless, a similar pattern seems to be developing. Side effects include menstrual problems, weight gain, headaches and depression. Particularly controversial is the question of whether women become more susceptible to breast cancer if they use injected contraceptives. Animal evidence suggests they will, but it is too early to make any definite judgment on human figures. The greatest disadvantage of a contraceptive injection from the user's point of view is that its effects continue for some months and cannot be reversed; infertility may last for much longer than expected.

14.11 ALTERNATIVES TO DRUGS FOR CONTRACEPTION

Most of the reliable alternative forms of contraception are well known: the condom, the diaphragm, the intrauterine device (IUD) and sterilization. Other methods of "natural contraception," such as the rhythm method ("Vatican roulette"), have a very high failure rate.

Both the condom and the diaphragm are returning to popularity as women become disenchanted with the Pill. Used with care they can be very effective, and they have the additional advantage of offering some protection from sexually transmitted infection. Using a condom significantly reduces the risk of contracting AIDS. You have to allow yourself time to grow accustomed to them, as initially they may seem awkward. If you are considering a diaphragm, go to your local contraception clinic. They have experience and a range of products so they can choose the right one for you. It is essential to use a spermicide with a diaphragm; you will be given cream and pessaries when you are fitted.

Spermicides used without a condom or diaphragm (including C-film, which can get dislodged or may not adequately cover the cervix) are not reliable forms of contraception. They offer some protection but you really do need a physical barrier to prevent those sperm from swimming rapidly up the cervix away from the poisons. New methods are being developed, but you should look for reliable evidence of effectiveness before you put your trust in some product bought over the drugstore counter.

The IUD seems to suit some women, particularly those who have had babies. It is very reliable and you don't have to think about it once it is fitted. Unfortunately it may bring itself to your attention by causing pain. If you get a lot of pain, have it removed; it can set up a pelvic infection from which you may never fully recover. Pelvic inflammatory disease (PID) may leave you infertile through damage to the fallopian tubes. The risk of this painful condition is much higher if you have an IUD inserted. If you have ever suffered from PID, don't let anybody talk you into having another IUD fitted; the chances are that you will just go through the same miserable process again.

Sterilization is by far the most satisfactory option for those who are confident they are not going to want more children. Once you have recovered from the operation you won't feel any different; you just won't have to worry about pregnancy ever again.

Vasectomy (male sterilization) is a simpler operation than the female equivalent, and couples would be wise to choose this option. It has no known long-term adverse effects; it does not affect the man's sex drive nor his ability to satisfy a woman. All it does is disconnect the tube which carries the sperm. Even the semen is produced as usual; it just does not contain any sperm. Vasectomy is a good method even for couples who are not absolutely certain that they will never want a baby because it is possible to put semen on ice in a sperm bank and draw on it when needed.

Female sterilization once caused lasting problems to some women through damage to their internal organs, but this is not true of the technique used today. The doctor will fit your fallopian tubes with tiny nylon rings or similar devices so that they do not allow the egg through. The operation can be done with a local anesthetic; you walk into a clinic, get sterilized through two tiny cuts in your abdomen, and walk out shortly afterward.

14.12 INFERTILITY

Almost one couple in seven in developed countries is infertile, and the number is growing. The older you are the less fertile you become; one British study showed that three quarters of women who become pregnant at the age of thirty have had unprotected intercourse for over two years before they conceive.

There are many reasons for infertility; damage to a woman's pelvic organs caused by infection is common, especially in those who have used an IUD. The Pill delays the return of ovulation in about 2% of women. Exposure to drugs (including alcohol and cigarettes) and chemicals can reduce fertility in both men and women, as can a poor diet high in additives and low in essential nutrients. Psychological problems and the couple's sexual behavior are also important (see section 14.14).

14.13   DRUGS FOR INFERTILITY

Hormone treatment is occasionally given to selected infertile women to induce ovulation. However, when failure of ovulation is not the cause of the problem, this treatment is inappropriate. The main problem with it is that it can cause multiple pregnancy. Hormone treatment is occasionally given to men whose sperm production is faulty, but this is a rare cause of infertility.

14.14   ALTERNATIVES TO DRUGS FOR INFERTILITY

(a) Diet and chemical intake

Both partners should aim to build up their general level of nutrition and to cut down their intake of chemicals in food. Not only will this increase the chance of conception but is also likely to enhance the health of the baby. (See section 18.2.)

Zinc supplements may be helpful for the infertile man but these should not be necessary if he eats plenty of organically produced food (see section 18.4(j)).

Try to give up all drugs, whatever their form. This includes both recreational drugs and medicines.

Certain industrial and domestic substances, as well as many pesticides, are capable of damaging sperm. The testis is very sensitive to chemicals. If you are exposed to high levels of chemicals in your work, you should consider changing your job. Infertility is just one of many possible health consequences of exposure to a high chemical load.

See also section 14.8; even if a woman is still having periods, hormone upsets can inhibit ovulation.

(b) Sexual behavior

Some inexperienced couples are infertile because they do not have intercourse correctly. If there is any possibility that you might have the mechanics of sex wrong—a surprising number of people do—get a manual such as Alex Comfort's *The Joy of Sex* and go through it together. Consult a counselor if you are uncertain or unhappy about your sex life.

The best time for conception is during ovulation, usually twelve to fourteen days after the beginning of the woman's period. Many women feel a heightened sex drive at this time. You can chart ovulation using a thermometer; the woman should take her temperature first thing in the morning (before the first drink) and watch for a half-degree rise in temperature. When this happens she is likely to be most fertile.

If you have intercourse every day or more often there may be few sperm available each time. You will improve the chances of conception by making love on alternate days. Intercourse should end with the man's climax; finish with the woman underneath and on her belly (doggy-fashion). After intercourse the woman should remain lying facedown for a while to give the sperm the best chance of swimming into her uterus.

A man who wishes to maximize his fertility should avoid tight trousers, tight underpants, hot baths and saunas. Sperm prefer a cool environment; this is why the testes hang outside the body in a skin bag.

If you make love rarely you might miss the crucial days when the woman is fertile. Make sure you have intercourse in the middle of the menstrual month. Consult a marriage counselor if you are not enjoying sex together enough to want to do it more often; this is usually a symptom of deeper relationship difficulties which could cause serious problems if a baby does arrive, stressing the relationship still further.

(c) Stress

Stress is a potent inhibitor of ovulation in women and sperm formation in men. Use the information in chapter 16 to deal more effectively with stress in your life. Ironically, the intensity of your desire for a baby can be enough to prevent conception! Previously infertile women quite frequently become pregnant after giving up the struggle and adopting.

If the problem is caused by stress, remember that nature is working on your behalf. A baby would add to your stress load and that would not be good for any of you. Look at your life as a whole: can you make significant changes that would reduce the pressure on you? Perhaps you would have to accept a lower standard of living, or life in a less stimulating environment. What sacrifices are you able or willing to make for the sake of a baby? Have you really confronted that question, or is your body perhaps protecting you by preventing the conflict?

Few would-be parents are fully aware of the enormous drain on energy and financial resources that a baby represents, and many parents regret having children without thinking it through thoroughly first. Our culture views the prospect of children through a romantic haze, and the media glorify motherhood, yet many of the problems faced by parents can be directly attributed to the fact that they had families when they were unable to support them financially or emotionally. If you never have children you will have many other opportunities to enrich your life. Infertility can be a boon—if you allow yourself to see it that way.

14.15 VAGINAL AND VULVAL ITCHING AND SORENESS (VAGINITIS)

Vaginitis and vulvovaginitis mean irritation of the vagina and the area around its entrance. The soreness and itching are often accompanied by increased discharge from the vagina. This pattern of symptoms can be due to a number of causes, some of which may occur together. Judge by the color and smell of your discharge whether you should consult a doctor to get a diagnosis of the problem; treatment is not always necessary and you should try self-care first. However, if the discharge smells revolting and is very different from normal, it is probably due to infection which will require medical treatment.

Part of the broad approach to preventing vaginitis is to maintain a state of optimum immunity by eating well and living a well-balanced life, though there are more specific measures you can use to enhance the health of the genital area.

Vaginitis often occurs when women are under stress or when they are suffering from other forms of illness, and it has become more common over recent years. One of the causes is the way we "clean" and dress ourselves. Chemical irritation by soaps, deodorants, disinfectants and detergents makes us more susceptible; wearing pantyhose, panties and trousers made of synthetic fibers that do not allow the genital area to breathe compounds the problem.

If you suffer from any form of vaginal irritation, be sure that only natural fabrics cover your crotch; cotton is best. Change your underwear frequently, washing it with pure soap if possible and rinsing thoroughly in soft water so that no residue is left. Even the smallest quantity of most detergent powders—especially those that contain enzymes—can irritate the delicate openings of the vagina and urethra, making you vulnerable to infection.

Spermicidal pessaries, creams, foams and other products can cause vaginitis in sensitive people. Allergic reactions can also occur with medicinal pessaries. The timing of the irritation should allow you to pinpoint the culprit; once it is identified the solution is simple: stop using it. You may find that a slightly different form causes no problems; for example, some women find that spermicidal pessaries produce an unpleasant reaction while cream is fine.

Never allow any deodorant or perfumed product near your genital area. Bath salts, bubble baths and bath oils are not for women who tend to suffer from problems of this type; in fact, you would be wiser to shower because the soap you use on your body will be in your bathwater and it could irritate the vulva. Don't use talcum powder or sanitary products that contain "freshening" agents, and don't let your sexual partner introduce soap or any other potential irritant into you on an insufficiently rinsed penis, on dirty or chemically contaminated fingers or in any form of sex play.

When you use a lubricant in sexual activity make sure it is a product such as K-Y jelly which is designed specifically for the purpose. Other creams may cause irritation. Lubricants can reduce the risk of vaginitis especially in older women whose natural estrogen has fallen below the level necessary to keep the vagina moist. However, they are no substitute for proper sexual arousal.

If you have lubrication problems, first try more preliminary sex play; fantasy—perhaps an erotic novel or film—can also prepare your body for enjoyable sex. Women who passively accept sexual activity when they do not actually want it are setting up problems for themselves, of which vulvovaginitis is just the beginning. If this could be the real cause of your difficulty, make an appointment with a counselor.

Refined carbohydrates (foods prepared using white flour or any form of sugar) in the diet increase the risk of vulvovaginitis because sugary urine provides a more favorable environment for any hostile organism. And since organisms which can cause vaginitis live in the bowel, women should always wipe themselves from front to back after going to the bathroom. This is a very important lesson for all little girls.

Vaginitis is more likely when the vagina is less acid than normal, so you should aim to maintain the acidity of the area. Add a couple of tablespoons of distilled vinegar to the water you use to wash your genital area. Avoid all types of soap or cleanser; even if the brand you use contains no perfume, it will change the biological balance of your membranes.

If your vaginal area is sore from sexual activity, excessive bicycle riding or similar mechanical stress, soothe it by bathing in warm (not hot) salt water. Use about a teaspoon of sea salt to a pint of pure water and bathe the area gently and thoroughly.

Douching is not recommended. Whatever solution you use, you are likely to disrupt the biological balance of your vagina and reduce your resistance to infection. In the United States, where douching is popular, vaginitis due to bacteria is much more common than in Britain; it is believed that the two are linked. The only substance you should consider introducing into your vagina is live natural yogurt or yogurt starter; the lactobacillus in this is beneficial and protects against fungal infection (see section 14.18).

Some experts believe that women who are susceptible to vaginitis should not use tampons. However, sanitary napkins can rub and chafe, so choose the method of sanitary protection that is most comfortable for you. Change frequently, avoid products which contain deodorants, and avoid any form of applicator which causes discomfort or which may seem to scratch; in our view there is no justification for using tampon applicators at all.

14.16   Vaginal thrush (candidiasis)

A thick white curdy discharge associated with itching and soreness is the hallmark of thrush, the most common vaginal infection. It is caused by the fungus *Candida albicans* which lives in many parts of our bodies, usually harmlessly. Candida causes problems when it changes its form and begins to invade the mucous membranes. This occurs when the biological balance of the vagina is disturbed, or when the immune system is not functioning normally. Thrush can easily be diagnosed by a doctor, but regular sufferers will be able to identify it quite readily themselves.

Because thrush results from decreased resistance to organisms which are present in normal healthy women, it is more rational to deal with the reasons for the failure of resistance rather than simply attempting to kill the fungus.

14.17   Drugs for thrush

Vaginal thrush is usually treated with creams or pessaries which are inserted high into the vagina. Fungicidal products commonly used for this purpose include clotrimazole (Gyne-Lotrimin, Mycelex), miconazole (Monistat) and nystatin (Mycostatin, Nilstat). Fungicidal pessaries occasionally cause local irritation but have not been linked with any serious adverse effects. Some doctors prescribe tablets for people with recurring thrush problems, usually miconazole or nystatin. Side effects include nausea, vomiting, diarrhea and rashes.

The authoritative British doctors' reference book *The British National Formulary* introduces its section on antifungal drugs thus: "It is important to remember that fungal infections are frequently associated with a defect in host resistance which should, if possible, be corrected otherwise drug therapy may fail." In other words, drug treatment is no substitute for enhanced health.

14.18   ALTERNATIVES TO DRUGS FOR THRUSH

Oral contraceptives make many women more vulnerable to thrush. You can expect a general improvement in your health if you stop taking the Pill. Antibiotic treatment can also cause an outbreak of thrush because it kills the bacteria which keep the fungus under control. Never take antibiotics unless they are absolutely essential— usually they are not. You can partially counter this hazard by eating plenty of inactive natural yogurt to replace lost bacteria. Antibiotics in meat and chicken may contribute to the current thrush epidemic. Try to avoid ordinary butchers' or supermarket meat; buy organically reared meat from specialty stores or give up eating meat. Fish is fine.

In the event of an attack of thrush you must act quickly. Home methods of dealing with it may not work once the infection is well established. This is what you do when the itching begins: Scrub a large basin clean of detergent and other chemical residues. Fill with cool water to which you have added distilled vinegar (about two tablespoons to the gallon). Squat over your basin and wash the vulval area carefully and thoroughly with clean fingers (no flannel, no scrubbing). Pat dry with a clean towel. Then wipe the area with pure olive oil. Live natural yogurt inserted into the vagina (on a tampon if you like) will set up a population of lactobacilli which will control the yeast. Repeat this procedure night and morning.

Wear a skirt and stockings or loose cotton trousers. Give up pantyhose, panties, tights and tight trousers until all symptoms have gone. Build up your defenses against fungal infection by following the dietary advice in section 18.6 and by checking section 5.12.

14.19 OTHER VAGINAL INFECTIONS

A foamy, evil-smelling, yellow-green discharge is characteristic of *Trichomonas* ("trich"), another common cause of vaginitis. Trich is sexually transmitted, so your partner(s) will require treatment too. Other foul-smelling discharges are symptoms of infection by a range of organisms; many of these are also sexually transmitted, and some can cause serious damage. If you have such a discharge, and especially if you have pelvic pain, you should consult a doctor without delay. VD clinics attached to large hospitals are much better equipped to diagnose and treat problems of this sort than general practitioners. In general these clinics are friendly and efficient, and your local one should be your first port of call if you develop a nasty vaginal discharge.

Once you have symptoms of vaginal or pelvic infection by bacteria or similar organisms, you and your partner will require drug therapy. There is no alternative. Similarly, there is no alternative to medical therapy for vaginal warts; get them treated quickly and thoroughly because they have been linked with cervical cancer. After such treatment, make sure you have regular cervical smears; cervical cancer can be cured if caught early. Reduce your vulnerability to genital infection by taking the following precautions:

1. Look very coolly and carefully at the genitalia of any new sexual partner. If you see a sore or anything that looks unhealthy, refuse contact until it has been investigated. Make sure the man has washed thoroughly, especially under the foreskin, and rinsed all soap residues away.
2. Insist that an unfamiliar sexual partner, or any man who has other lovers, wear a condom. This is your best protection against AIDS, which is becoming increasingly common among heterosexuals, and against other sexually transmitted disease.
3. Don't use an IUD (intrauterine device, or coil). The chances of

infection are much higher in IUD users, and it can result in pelvic inflammatory disease (PID)—a most painful condition which may leave you sterile.

14.20 HERPES

Like thrush, herpes is caused by an organism that is very widespread but which produces symptoms only when there is some defect in your resistance. Genital herpes is usually caught during intercourse or oral sex with a sufferer who has active sores on the lips or genitals; symptoms begin two to twelve days after infection. The cause is a virus (*Herpes simplex*) which is shed from the sores and which then lives in the body. However, herpes is a hardy virus which can survive on a wide range of surfaces—from toilet seats to wrestling mats—so it may not be possible to avoid contact with it.

The virus cannot be eliminated from your body once it has taken up residence, and you may never know about it because it may cause no symptoms if you are healthy. Normally, symptoms flare up when your resistance is low. The first attack is usually the worst; the symptoms diminish in severity with time as the body builds up immunity to the virus. The average person will not have more than six recurrences.

During a herpes attack, sufferers develop numerous tiny blisters on the membranes of the vagina or penis and genital areas, and often on the skin of the thighs and around the anus. These blisters burst, turning into ulcers which are extremely tender. Any irritant—including urine—will cause pain; intercourse may be agonizing and must be completely avoided. The lymph glands in the groin swell, and you may suffer fever and headache. After a week or so the symptoms disappear spontaneously.

14.21 DRUGS FOR HERPES

No drug currently available is capable of getting rid of herpes infection and preventing recurrence. A new product, acyclovir (Zovirax), can reduce the severity of an attack, but because it is new, some of its effects and potential hazards will not yet be known. Zovirax can be taken in tablet form or used on the lesions themselves. Adverse effects include metabolic changes and rashes. Reduce the risk of these by drinking large amounts of water.

14.22 ALTERNATIVES TO DRUGS FOR HERPES

The development of symptoms of herpes and the length of time an attack lasts both depend on the immune status of the sufferer. The best way of coping with it is to do all you can to increase your overall immunity to infection (see section 5.12). Good nutrition (see chapter 18) and adequate rest are crucial.

Stress plays an important role in herpes. Deal with emotional stress by embarking on one or more of the strategies described in chapter 16.

If you have an outbreak of herpes, don't share it with those around you by sharing clothes or towels. Avoid spreading it to new sites on your own body by washing very thoroughly after touching yourself anywhere near the infected area; the sores produce a watery discharge that contains many active viruses, and you must be sure to scrub this off your hands if there is any possibility that they have become contaminated.

Women should deal with the discomfort of genital herpes as with other forms of vaginitis (see section 14.15). Tampons and sanitary napkins may be irritating if you have herpes and a period at the same time. Try using a disposable napkin inside loose panties. Painful urination can be relieved with cool water. Try urinating in a shower.

Try daubing Milk of Magnesia on your sores; it will relieve pain. Do not shake the bottle but let it stand until the liquid separates. Pour the thin fluid off the top and use a long cotton swab to dip into the bottom of the bottle.

Witch hazel will help to dry up the ulcers. Get it from your pharmacist.

Lesions around the anal region cause pain when emptying the bowels. Keep the stools soft and loose by eating a whole-food diet (see sections 18.2 and 18.3) and drinking more pure water.

Finally, a very important warning for women who have suffered from genital herpes: *the herpes virus may cause cervical cancer.* You should have a cervical smear every year after your first attack—and make sure you get told the result. Cervical cancer is totally and readily curable if it is treated early.

14.23 INFECTIONS OF THE PENIS

The male sexual organs are far less likely to cause trouble than the female equivalent. However, the penis can be infected by fungal and other organisms; these may cause problems not only for the man but for his sexual partner(s). If you find a sore or wart on your penis, or if there is pain or any discharge, you should go to a VD clinic without delay. There are no alternatives to medical treatment for most of the infections that cause symptoms of this sort.

Soreness is not always associated with infection, however. If it is due to overuse, it can be soothed by bathing the penis frequently in cool salt water. Soreness under the foreskin is usually due to lack of hygiene. Wash very thoroughly with the foreskin drawn well back; soap is not necessary, but if you do use it, rinse all the residue away.

A slight rash under the foreskin and a curdy deposit may mean you have a fungal infection. Use a cream such as Mycelex or Lotrimin (available from the pharmacist), and add a tablespoon of vinegar to the water in which you wash your penis. If you have any difficulty in drawing the foreskin back completely, consult your doctor; he will be able to refer you to get it loosened or removed. Thorough, frequent and regular washing under the foreskin, or getting it removed, is essential if you want to please the ladies in your life. Women suffer the effects of an unhygienic penis because of its association with an increased risk of cervical cancer.

14.24 IMPOTENCE

Impotence is the inability to produce or maintain an erection sufficient for penetration and sexual intercourse. Although male hormones are occasionally prescribed for impotence, drug therapy is rarely appropriate and rarely used.

The most common causes of impotence fall into two groups: psychological problems and drugs. If you are taking any drugs, particularly drugs for cardiovascular problems, they could be the reason for your impotence. Ask your pharmacist if this effect is known with your medication, or look it up in the *Physicians' Desk Reference,* which is available in reference libraries. Alcohol is well known for its ability to induce impotence. Do you have a drinking problem?

Psychological causes of impotence include stress from any source and specific anxiety about sexual performance. If you have a lot of worries, if you have problems getting to sleep, or if you are depressed, study chapters 4 and 16 to learn ways of coping more effectively. You won't need to pay any special attention to the question of impotence; your potency is likely to return quite naturally when you are feeling better.

Anxiety about sex can readily induce impotence. Are you afraid that you will not be able to meet your partner's demands? Or perhaps you are ashamed of your sexuality? Maybe you don't really like your partner or you feel angry with her; emotions of this sort can readily result in impotence. Seek a counselor if you feel this is true in your case.

Certain types of illness can also cause impotence. Diabetes is becoming an increasingly frequent cause. It can produce temporary impotence through blood sugar fluctuations (a snack is likely to cure it if the diabetic is normally able to sustain an erection) or permanent disability through damage to the blood and nerve supply to the penis. Diabetics can do much to avoid this sort of damage by good health practices which reduce the severity of their illness (see section 10.4).

If you have suddenly become impotent and you cannot see any likely cause in your relationship or other aspects of your life, you would be wise to consult a doctor; it might be a symptom of illness which requires treatment.

15

Pregnancy and Birth

To many women the health of their babies is even more important than their own health, but the key to an uneventful pregnancy and the birth of a strong, healthy baby is for the mother to keep herself in top condition. The more you are able to maintain your health, the less you will need any form of medical help.

SECTION INDEX

15.1   Preparing for pregnancy
15.2   A healthy pregnancy
15.3   Illness during pregnancy
15.4   Drugs in pregnancy
15.5   Alternatives to drugs for problems of pregnancy
15.6   The medicalization of birth
15.7   Preparation for the birth
15.8   Starting labor
15.9   Labor and birth
15.10   Breast-feeding

15.1 PREPARING FOR PREGNANCY

Preparation for pregnancy should ideally begin months before you start trying for a baby. Your physical condition before conception has an important bearing on the future well-being of your baby. During pregnancy your body has to provide a full complement of nutrients for the development of the baby and the placenta that feeds it. In order to be sure that these will be plentiful when they are needed you must have good stores of nutrients in your tissues.

If you have recently had a baby, your body's stores of essential nutrients could still be low. It is wise to try to space your pregnancies out so that your body has ample opportunity to replenish these stores. Use barrier contraceptive methods to avoid conceiving for at least nine months after the last birth (see section 14.11). Don't continue taking the Pill if you want to have a baby within a year or so; your fertility may take some time to return, and in addition the Pill depletes your body's stores of nutrients. Give it up well in advance and use a cap or condom until you are ready to conceive.

Dieting is even more than usually foolish at this time. Indeed, statistics reveal that women who are overweight by the standards of our society have a markedly better chance of giving birth to healthy babies than those who are very slim when they conceive. Women who are underweight before pregnancy are four times as likely to have underweight babies; and underweight babies are many times more likely than those of normal weight to be spastic, to suffer from conditions ranging from spina bifida and heart malformations to persistent colds and breathing problems, and to die prematurely. So you should eat enough to ensure that you have a well-rounded body; you may think that slenderness looks good, but it won't be good for your baby.

If you are of average height (5′4″) your baby is most likely to be healthy if you weigh about 140 pounds before pregnancy—which is 20 pounds more than most women imagine they should weigh. But don't eat chocolate or sugary foods to gain weight; go for an organic whole food diet (see section 18.2) supplemented with extra nuts and fruit so that your flesh is of the highest quality. Eating a poor-quality diet, one that is high in refined sugar and white flour products and low in vitamins, trace minerals and micronutrients, reduces your body's ability to detoxify the chemicals that abound in our environment. Some of these are known to damage the genetic code. Not only can the woman and the eggs she carries be affected, but also the man's sperm production is very sensitive to the effects of toxins. So in the year before you intend to become pregnant you should ensure that you eat well and that you avoid exposing yourself and your partner to potential poisons. Give up smoking well before you become pregnant and make sure he does the same.

B-group vitamins (see sections 18.4(b) and 18.4(d)) are especially important both before and during pregnancy. The prevalence of birth defects in Scotland and Ireland, among the highest in the developed world, has been convincingly linked with a diet deficient in fresh green vegetables and whole grains which would provide these essential vitamins. Scottish and Irish women eat less of these crucial foods than the women of any other country in the Western world.

If you are thinking of trying for a baby, you should do all you can to try to get off all drugs *before* you conceive. By drugs we mean not just medication but also nicotine, alcohol and oral contraceptives. Obviously this is not always possible, but by following the advice in this book you may be able to reduce your need for them. It is worth making conscientious efforts to reduce your use of all medication because research has shown that women taking drugs for some types of chronic illness are more likely to give birth to handicapped children. Medication for epilepsy is a case in point, and the use of antiepileptic drugs can often be reduced.

15.2 A HEALTHY PREGNANCY

It should come as no surprise that the guiding principles for health during pregnancy are just the same as at other times. A balanced life, with activity and adequate rest when required; a balanced wholefood diet; a positive attitude to life, yourself and your growing baby; and the avoidance of environmental and dietary poisons will all give you and your baby the best possible chance of health.

(a) Diet

The levels of vitamins and minerals in your diet need to be higher during pregnancy because the developing baby requires these nutrients. Your doctor may prescribe supplements of iron and folic acid, though we believe that iron in the form of supplements can do more harm than good. Check section 18.4(*i*) for good dietary sources of iron. Folic acid and pyridoxine (vitamin B$_6$) are very important, and supplements containing small doses of these vitamins will do you no harm; but do also make sure you eat the foods that contain them (sections 18.4(*d*) and 18.4(*e*)).

Never take megadose vitamin tablets, and never try to substitute supplements for good eating habits. Megadoses could damage you and your baby and throw your body into imbalance. Be especially careful not to take tablets containing high doses of vitamins A and D, and don't take more than 50 mg. per day of pyridoxine. Get your vitamin A from carrots, fish and free-range eggs, and vitamin D from sunshine.

Many women (and some of their doctors) are concerned lest they put on too much weight during pregnancy. This preoccupation led to a vogue for food restriction. This is dangerous for babies. It is far more important to be sure that you are eating enough highly nutritious food than to limit weight gain. Indeed, statistics show that women who gain more weight during pregnancy are also likely to have healthier babies.

Try to cut your intake of both salt (section 18.12) and sugar (section 18.11). Avoiding sugar and sweet drinks will protect you from diabetes, which often develops during pregnancy, while restricting your salt intake will reduce the risk of high blood pressure and toxemia of pregnancy.

Drink plenty of fluid—six pints a day is sensible—especially pure bottled or filtered water and fruit juice. Avoid tea, coffee and soft drinks, and be wary about milk since it can induce allergies in your baby. If you like milk, choose skim and restrict yourself to a maximum of half a pint a day. Natural yogurt seems not to cause these problems for most people; the beneficial bacteria in yogurt apparently counter the potential hazard of the milk. Make sure the yogurt you eat is the genuine live form and not a processed substitute. Yogurt is particularly valuable late in pregnancy; it is a good source of calcium, which you need to build your baby's bones and to prepare your own body for breast-feeding.

Slight water retention, causing puffiness in the legs which is especially obvious during hot weather, is nothing to worry about. In fact, Swedish research has revealed that mothers who retain some water often have healthier babies.

(b) Activity

Pregnancy should not prevent you from enjoying any physical activity, though your size in late pregnancy will obviously limit you. Women who habitually go running and continue to do so during pregnancy tend to have easier births and healthy babies. And sexual activity poses no risk to your baby; indeed, by keeping you happy it is likely to be beneficial.

15.3   ILLNESS DURING PREGNANCY

If you develop an infection—even a minor one like a cold—during pregnancy you should increase your vitamin intake. As soon as you start to feel unwell, eat lots of oranges, fresh strawberries and other foods containing vitamin C (see section 18.4(f)). Also take supplements of B-group vitamins (section 18.4(b))—yeast tablets are very good—and try to get more fresh green vegetables (cabbage and broccoli rather than lettuce).

15.4   DRUGS IN PREGNANCY

Ever since the thalidomide tragedy it has been well known that drugs taken during pregnancy can damage the developing baby. Such damage can take many forms. A few drugs, known as mutagens, are capable of causing mutations in the genetic code which lead to wide-ranging and incurable disabilities; others such as thalidomide are teratogens capable of interfering with normal development; still others can increase your child's susceptibility to cancers. These are gross and dreadful effects, but drugs may also cause subtle damage such as behavior problems in the children of mothers who take certain painkillers or drugs that affect the mind during pregnancy. And we can be quite sure that the full range of such problems is not yet known and may never be acknowledged by some experts.

The mother and her baby are connected by the placenta, which carries the mother's blood supply and brings it into contact with her baby's circulation. Regrettably, the placenta seems to be incapable of protecting the baby from drugs and poisons in the mother's blood; these reach the baby along with the nutrients required for growth. The baby's liver works in tandem with the mother's to deal with chemicals, so if you are exposed to such substances your baby could be born with a damaged or highly stressed liver. Substances that are bad for the mother are likely to be even worse for the baby. Addictive drugs set up addiction in the womb; hospitals in major cities are now all too familiar with babies damaged by fetal alcohol syndrome and the tragedy of newborn heroin addicts going cold turkey in the nursery.

Alcohol is dangerous to the developing fetus during the first three months of pregnancy. Thereafter, light social drinking may do no harm unless your body is not readily able to metabolize alcohol. So judge whether you can enjoy the occasional drink by your reaction to alcohol before pregnancy. If you suffered badly from hangovers, don't drink; if you were fine except when you really overindulged, your body probably copes quite well with alcohol. But do avoid it right at the end of pregnancy when the birth could be imminent, because alcohol slows down labor.

During the first few weeks of pregnancy, the cells of the fetus are dividing rapidly and differentiating into the various types of tissue and organ. At this stage drugs can interfere with the accuracy of development by disrupting a critical period of morphogenesis—the development of the form of the new baby. Sometimes this critical time is very clear-cut; thalidomide was found to be relatively harmless during most of pregnancy, but if a woman took a single tablet on the fortieth day, her baby was almost certain to be born deformed.

It is tragically true that drugs assumed to be perfectly safe for both mother and child at the time they are administered may later be shown to have horrific dangers, and sometimes, that drugs which are known to be dangerous are nevertheless given to pregnant women. Sex hormones prescribed to prevent habitual miscarriage have been linked with a wide range of malformations. One synthetic sex hormone, DES (diethylstilbestrol), was found to cause vaginal cancers in the daughters of women who were treated with the drug during pregnancy, and serious problems with the sex organs of their sons. DES is no longer used, and many other similar products have now been withdrawn, but synthetic sex hormones are still being given to pregnant women despite the fact that there is no evidence that they have any value. If miscarriage has been your problem do *not* accept medication; follow instead the advice in this chapter.

Even some of the most commonly used drugs can damage your baby. Aspirin, tranquilizers and sleeping tablets are among those that have been found to increase the chances of malformation. Aspirin taken during the last few weeks of pregnancy increases the risk of hemorrhage by mother and baby at the time of the birth. It should be avoided throughout pregnancy. Some laxatives may be hazardous during pregnancy; if you eat enough vegetables, fruit and whole grains you will never have any need for them.

The *British National Formulary* includes a long list of drugs that should be avoided during pregnancy. Almost every type of drug is included in the list, and the editors warn that "the absence of a drug from this list does not imply safety."

(a) Drugs for morning sickness

This is a controversial area. Court cases have been fought over deformities claimed to be due to the drug Bendectin. Parents of children alleged to be damaged continue to fight for compensation. The medical establishment has not accepted that drugs for morning sickness are dangerous but Bendectin has been withdrawn. According to the *British National Formulary*, drugs are not generally required.

(b) *Drugs for high blood pressure*

It is not unusual for pregnant women to develop high blood pressure, and a range of antihypertensive drugs may be prescribed to reduce the risk to the baby that this entails. In this situation drugs are seen as the lesser hazard, but the best answer is to do everything possible to prevent the development of high blood pressure so that medication never becomes necessary. See sections 9.10 and 9.11 for information on those drugs and their alternatives.

15.5 ALTERNATIVES TO DRUGS FOR PROBLEMS OF PREGNANCY

Good nutrition and adequate relaxation throughout pregnancy are the best ways of avoiding any need for drugs. If you suffer badly from morning sickness, try eating dry toast or rice cakes. Experiment with plain foods until you find something you can keep down. Iron tablets sometimes cause nausea, so if you are taking them try stopping for a while and eating more iron-rich foods like dark green leafy vegetables and dark meat (18.4(i)). Supplement your diet with 50 mg. per day of vitamin B_6. But do try not to get unduly worried by morning sickness; it will pass, and it does not mean your baby is at risk.

Threatened miscarriage should be treated with rest, relaxation and a good diet—not with drugs. The most risky months are the third and fourth; if you have had miscarriages in the past you should take things very easy at this time. Get in a stock of good reading and put your feet up.

15.6 THE MEDICALIZATION OF BIRTH

The medicalization of birth—treating birth like an illness rather than as a natural healthy event—has led to a high level of drug use for birth. Medical assumptions about how to cope with labor have tended to lead to excessive intervention and unnecessary pain, and the rising rate of births by cesarian section is a disturbing trend.

A wide range of medical measures is used to "assist" birth. These range from hormones, given to induce labor, to potent anesthetics. After a period in the 1970s when intervention was ubiquitous, the medical profession is now interfering less and women and their babies are faring better. Nevertheless, many obstetricians still use drugs far more often than critics think they should.

Drugs given to the mother during labor undoubtedly affect her baby. The recent vogue for induction of a very high proportion of births was linked directly with an epidemic of neonatal jaundice. The baby's immature liver is not able to deal efficiently with drugs and hormones, and jaundice is one result of this. Babies often suffer breathing difficulties when their mothers are given painkilling drugs during labor; induced babies are particularly prone to this.

In ideal circumstances the baby would not be exposed to any drugs during birth. This is the aim of the natural-childbirth movement. However, it may be that all your efforts are insufficient to prevent severe pain, and you should not feel distressed if you need drugs for pain relief. The best you can aim for is to minimize your chances of needing drugs by preparing as well as you can for the birth.

15.7 PREPARATION FOR THE BIRTH

Breathing and relaxation classes to prepare you for the birth are available all over the country. The methods taught in these classes help enormously with labor, and many women find that they also prove valuable for stress relief in subsequent years. Contact the Childbirth Without Pain Association, 20134 Snowden, Detroit, MI 48235, (313) 341–3816, for information about natural ways of preventing pain.

Learn as much as possible about childbirth well in advance of the event. Sheila Kitzinger's *The Experience of Childbirth* is excellent, but there are many other books in this area. Try to get your partner to read and learn about it; it is best if fathers go to birth preparation classes too, so that they know how they can help their partners to cope. If men are not welcome at the classes to which you were planning to go, look around for classes which you can both attend.

If you are able to have your baby at home you will be exposed to far fewer drugs and far less medical intervention than if the birth takes place in a hospital. In hospitals over 90% of mothers are given drugs for pain relief during labor, and it is often impossible for the mother to avoid them. Comparisons with other countries show that drugs are neither necessary nor desirable; in the Netherlands only 5% of mothers need pain-relieving drugs, and nearly half the babies are born at home. The figures for perinatal mortality (death of the mother or baby in birth or during the first year thereafter) reveal that the countries with low levels of drug use are also the safest for both mother and child. In Scandinavia and the Netherlands perinatal mortality is at about half the U.S. level.

Recent figures show clearly that home is, overall, the safest place to have your baby. If it is your second or third baby, if you are in good health and you have not had any real difficulties in the past (apart from those caused directly by medical intervention), you might be wise to consider a home confinement. Contact the American College of Home Obstetrics, P.O. Box 25, River Forest, IL 60305, (312) 383-1461, if you do not know a doctor who is happy about attending home births. Information and support for home births is also available from the International Association for Childbirth at Home, P.O. Box 39498, Los Angeles, CA 90039, (213) 667-0839. However, you will find it particularly difficult to persuade doctors to agree to a home birth if it is your first baby and there is anything less than ideal about your home (for example, if there is nobody to look after you, or if you have no convenient bathroom), if you are over thirty-five, or if you have a very small build. Don't expect to have subsequent babies at home if you have had any previous problems with childbirth (such as a stillbirth, hemorrhage or Cesarian). If you have health problems such as diabetes, or kidney, respiratory or heart disease, you will be expected to have all your babies in the hospital.

If you are considering a home birth we recommend Sheila Kitzinger's *Birth at Home*.

15.8 STARTING LABOR

You should be very reluctant to allow your labor to be started artificially. Induced babies are not generally as healthy as those that are born after a natural labor, and the pain caused to the mother is considerably greater.

Induction is associated with an increased need for epidural anesthesia; this interferes with the mother's ability to control the birth so that forceps delivery is more likely to be necessary. In addition, the baby's head may be compressed during an induced birth and this could cause brain damage. There are also problems in the mother's relationship with the baby after induction, primarily because of the level of anesthesia required; an induced birth is a much less joyful event than a natural one.

Some obstetricians believe in inducing labor when a baby is thought to be a week or so late; in fact, many of these babies are not late at all. If your obstetrician advises induction, you should raise questions about it. Find out exactly why he suggests it. Don't allow yourself to be pressured; try to get a second opinion. But do acknowledge that he could be right; when the baby really is at risk through continued pregnancy, induction makes sense.

If your baby does seem to be late, and the obstetrician is pressing, see if you can induce labor naturally. Use sex to increase your body's production of labor-inducing oxytocin; extended sexual arousal and orgasms could do the trick. Nipple stimulation is helpful, particularly if it makes you sexually excited.

It is very important that you *drink no alcohol.* This will slow down the birth. Also, *don't take aspirin;* it could cause hemorrhage.

15.9 LABOR AND BIRTH

At your prenatal classes you should have learned the techniques on which you will depend to control labor and birth and to reduce your need for any pain-reducing medication. It cannot be stressed too heavily that these classes are very important to new mothers. The details of the breathing and relaxation methods are not readily understood from a book; you must take lessons from a competent teacher.

The information given below assumes that you have a lot of choice about where you are and what you can do. If you are not having your baby at home, where you would have maximum freedom, it is worth-while choosing a hospital where you will be allowed to move about as you wish. This will give you the best chance of controlling any pain you experience. In addition, the sort of place that respects your desire to choose your most comfortable position and be active in the birth is less likely to foist unwanted drugs upon you.

Once labor has begun you should try to stay on your feet for as long as possible; women who walk around while in labor suffer less pain. Do light housework or gardening, dance to records, take a stroll, entertain your friends. If you feel sleepy, though, lie down for a snooze; you have hard work ahead! Soak in a warm bath. Eat a light meal with your partner (an omelet, yogurt and banana, or sand-wiches).

If you suffer from backache during labor, ask your husband or helper to rub your back, using firm pressure from the heel of the hand or knuckles. A hot-water bottle on the sore area may help. Experi-ment with your position; you may be more comfortable on all fours (playing Scrabble on the floor?) or kneeling forward supported by beanbags or large floor cushions.

During each contraction breathe slowly in at the beginning and slowly out at the end. If necessary take some light, quick breaths at the crest of the contraction, but be careful not to breathe too fast for more than a few seconds, as that is liable to make you feel unneces-sarily anxious and distressed. As contractions become more frequent (every two to three minutes) you will need to relax completely between each one. By this time you should aim to be at the place where you are going to have your baby. If you are at home your partner should call the midwife if he has not already done so. This is when you will be drawing on what you learned during classes. Con-centrate on your breathing; you should know the technique so well that it is automatic. Focus your eyes on your partner's face or the window. Relax your shoulders. Your partner may be able to help by sponging you with cold water or massaging your inner thighs. Ask for whatever you feel will help.

In the final stages of labor you are likely to be offered analgesia. Continue to experiment with your position; giving birth lying on your back is likely to be considerably more difficult than squatting.

Controlled breathing is very important, as is relaxation of all the parts of the body not involved in the birth effort. The right time to push is when you *want* to; do what comes naturally and trust your feelings.

When your baby is born it is time for cuddles, ecstatic joy, celebration! New mothers who have had no drugs feel very awake and acutely aware. It could be the happiest time of your whole life.

15.10   BREAST-FEEDING

Drugs taken by the mother almost always contaminate her breast milk. For this reason it is wise to continue to avoid all drugs during the period of breast-feeding. There is a risk that even when the quantity of drug in breast milk is very small it may be enough to cause hypersensitivity in the infant. With some drugs the concentration in breast milk is much higher than in the mother's blood, so the baby will receive a dangerously large dose.

If you require drugs for maintenance therapy of chronic illness, always try to keep doses as low as possible. Be aware that your responsiveness to your drugs may have changed after your baby's birth, so be especially sensitive to your own needs. Make sure your diet contains high levels of all the nutrients you need for effective liver function (see sections 18.5(a), 18.4(d), 18.4(f), and 18.4(i)).

Oral contraceptives can suppress the flow of milk; avoid them. Breast-feeding acts as a natural contraceptive, though it is not completely safe, so you would be wise to use a backup method such as the condom. Also, avoid common nonprescription drugs including aspirin which can cause rashes and adversely affect the baby's blood.

PART 3

HEALTH CHOICES

Introduction

MAKING positive choices involves change. Some changes will be minor and easy; others will be more profound and difficult, particularly if you live in a family. The best solution is to discuss with your family the health choices you plan to make, and take them with you. Everyone will benefit, though old habits, tastes and beliefs may provoke resistance.

You should be aware of the possible effects on your principal relationship. Change will affect you both, and patience and understanding may be required.

16

Stress Management

We are all affected by stress. It is part of the price we pay for living too close to other people, or too much apart from them; for getting too involved with the demands of modern society, or being too isolated from them; for being overstimulated, or being understimulated. In short, stress results when our lives are seriously out of balance.

Our reactions to stress are part of the coping mechanisms our body and mind have developed to help weather rough patches until the normal balance of things is restored. It is perfectly normal to react to difficulties with a bout of anxiety, an increase in blood pressure, or activity to the point of exhaustion, after which we return to a state of calm. Stress becomes a problem only when balance is not restored, when we try to live in a state where anxiety, high blood pressure or exhaustion is the norm.

Dealing with chronic stress is difficult, for although the symptoms may fall into several easily identified patterns, the causes do not. We vary enormously in our susceptibility and reactions to stress according to the many things which make up our individual being, the things we respond to and the values we hold in life.

There are no simple answers to stress problems. We each have to identify the causes and either remove or moderate them or increase our capacity to cope with them. Whatever the cause, the answer is likely to be fairly basic; you will have to get the basics right to have any worthwhile effect. No pill, no gadget, no tinkering with bad habits and no amount of self-delusion will have the same fundamental effect.

It is in dealing with chronic stress that the conventional medical approach of treating symptoms finally comes unstuck. For instance, it is quite clear that lowering blood pressure by giving drugs, without dealing with the reason for its increase, will simply transfer the stress reaction to another system in the body. Indeed, it will probably make things worse, as the body will have to cope not only with the original stress but also with the added stress caused by the disabling of one of its coping mechanisms. Trying to deal with stress by giving drugs is like trying to lower the temperature of a room by cooling the thermometer. It creates an unsatisfactory and potentially dangerous illusion.

Yet something needs to be done about the diseases related to stress. Heart and circulatory diseases are now the biggest killer in the world. In America 40% of all deaths are caused by heart disease, and chronic stress is a major contributor to this epidemic. Whereas these conditions used to be associated with old age, they are now creeping down the age scale; children are now found with hardening of the arteries, and fatal heart attacks in people in their thirties have become more common.

Other potentially fatal diseases in which chronic stress plays a significant part are ulcers, depression, cancer and asthma. Chronic stress also helps infections get a better grip, and this may prove fatal in debilitated individuals. Stress can induce disabling conditions such as insomnia, anxiety, ulcerative colitis, spastic colon, cystitis, backache and headache, and it can also bring on menstrual problems, infertility, infections and skin disorders.

Before leaving this general section, mention must be made of common things which are relevant to the stress problem—dieting *and smoking. People who habitually diet are imposing an unnecessary stress on themselves. Dieting is mostly a waste of effort since it does not work. Yes, you will lose weight initially—any change or metabolic shake-up will cause that—but in the end the weight goes on again. We would like you to repeat the motto* DIETING MAKES YOU FAT *until the truth sinks in. Eat naturally, balance food with rest and activity, and you can be whatever shape you wish without suffering. (See chapters 17 and 18.) Smokers who are under severe stress should not attempt to give up smoking until they have tackled the problem which reinforces their habit. If you use nicotine as a crutch, do not knock it away when it is still needed. But do not use this as a reason to continue smoking indefinitely.*

SECTION INDEX

16.1   *Recuperation*
16.2   *Exhaustion*
16.3   *Solutions to stress*
16.4   *The need for relaxation*
16.5   *Breathing*
16.6   *Relaxation methods*
16.7   *Preparing for sleep*
16.8   *Unwinding*
16.9   *Meditation*
16.10   *Yoga*
16.11   *Muscle relaxation*
16.12   *Breathing for panic attacks*
16.13   *Dealing with worry*
16.14   *Confidence*
16.15   *Counseling*
16.16   *Wider causes of stress*

16.1 RECUPERATION

When we are awake and active we use up energy and wear down our minds and bodies; when we are asleep we refill our energy stores, rebuild our tissues and clear our minds. When stimulated, the brain directs appropriate action; when the stimulation ends, the brain directs recuperation. If we are overstimulated, the time available for recuperation diminishes, the immune system becomes less efficient, energy stores run down and we depend on more stimulation, from drugs or adrenaline, to motivate us. A vicious circle is created. If we are in a high-pressure job or life-style, the overstimulation prevents recuperation and we slide into one of the many chronic disease patterns described on the previous page.

Working hard and playing hard are fine provided that they are balanced by adequate rest and recuperation. If they are not, you will find yourself sliding backwards. At first, perhaps borne along by youth and achievement, you may not notice, but sooner or later you will become a victim of some of the conditions ascribed to stress. Once you reach this point, trying harder will only accelerate your decline.

16.2 EXHAUSTION

Many people who suffer exhaustion do not recognize it for what it is. They continue with their daily grind, trapped by commitments, caught on the career ladder. Their stress load has become an integral part of their lives, and although they may be aware of the risks and the personal deterioration, they can see no way out. They continue to push themselves, they ignore the emerging symptoms of stress, and they finally arrive at a state of exhaustion.

If people continue struggling to work when they are exhausted, their efforts will achieve less and less. Failing energies will do more to damage them than to solve the problems they face. They will get into a position where they are unable to sleep and recover adequately. The

THE MALE FUNCTION CURVE

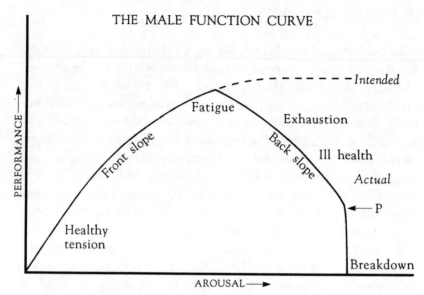

P represents the "catastrophic cliff edge" of instability where little further arousal is required to precipitate a breakdown.

Source: Nixon, P. "Stress and the Cardiovascular System."
The Practitioner 226 (1982): 1590.

only solution then is total rest and recuperation. The diagrams here and on page 272 show why this is the case.

The male function curve describes the relationship between effective performance and arousal (or stimulation). Healthy exertion occurs on the front of the curve where the level of arousal is not excessive. Living on the front slope of the function curve, people experience tension and fatigue on a cyclic basis.

Those who have passed beyond recuperation into exhaustion are living on the back slope. Typically they *believe* their performance is fine (on the intended line)—whereas actually it progressively declines. Living here leads to illness; if you are in this state when you go for that one final push of effort, you risk breakdown. At point P, this can be serious.

Cardiologist Peter Nixon, who developed the concept of the human function curve in relation to heart attack, explains it thus: "Life can easily become a battle to close the gap between what the individual actually can achieve and what he or she thinks is expected; the struggle is self-defeating, however, because the additional arousal pushes the individual inexorably downwards into illness."

The secret of avoiding breakdown is twofold. First, learn to recognize the signs of exhaustion and failing productivity, and stop working as soon as these emerge rather than carrying on with the help of coffee and other drugs. Second, you can try to increase your effective capacity by living a more balanced life, alternating striving with relaxation. By so doing you extend the length of your front slope. You become capable of much more without being forced into a state of exhaustion on that dangerous back slope.

Males are designed for steady output, with occasional bursts of high-energy activity—call them sprints. Modern life frequently demands that men sprint all the time, and those who cannot keep up without having to do this will suffer.

The female function curve is slightly more complicated. The diagram below refers to premenopausal women; after menopause the function curve is similar to the male's. We have shown two curves because female coping capacity varies widely according to hormone balance at any particular time. In the middle weeks of the menstrual month, high arousal may be associated with excellent function; but just before and during a period, high arousal can cause performance and energy to deteriorate much more quickly. Women need to recognize these fluctuations in capacity within themselves.

Women have more stamina than men; they may not be as strong or as fast in absolute terms but they are better designed for the long, steady haul. Generally they do not get led into the competitive situations which men create for themselves. In women, stress tends to emerge in anxiety, depression, autoimmune disease and cancer, rather than in the kind of catastrophic breakdown epitomized in the male by heart attack.

While women do suffer stress disease if they live on that long back slope, they are not as likely as men to suffer catastrophic breakdown. This capacity is built into the female to enable her to survive the

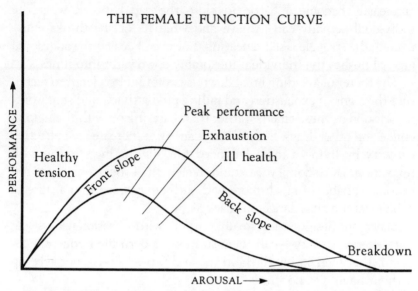

THE FEMALE FUNCTION CURVE

The function curve will vary with hormone state. Female physical endurance is not characterized by catastrophic failure. The decline from exhaustion to breakdown typically exhibits a range of types of illness.

extreme requirements of pregnancy, birth and child rearing. However, a capacity which enables survival is not the same as one in which a person will thrive. The answer for women is the same as for men: alternate striving and relaxation so that you increase the capacity of the front slope; living there and avoiding the hazardous back slope, you will maximize your capability and retain your health.

Warning: If you are exhausted, you must *not* attempt to increase your physical or coping capacity until you have learned how to relax and have spent some time, perhaps months, recuperating. If you feel you could sleep for a week, take time to do so.

16.3 SOLUTIONS TO STRESS

The ideal solution to the stress problem lies in the full use of our bodies and our minds. We need to be physically competent and take pleasure in our bodies and in the range of experiences available in the combination of mind and body. Today education avoids this connection; consequently people are incompetent in many crucial areas of life. Not only does this inhibit their capacity to live on the front slope of the function curve, but it is also a source of stress in itself.

Many of those who seek to enhance their health by taking up jogging can be seen waddling ineffectually around the park wasting most of their time and effort because they have never learned to move effectively. Many of those who do not make it to the park must be much worse. Without physical competence and a sense of joy in our being, we will not take pleasure in the use of our bodies. Without that basic pleasure, any attempt to increase physical capacity will involve a battle with ourselves which we will usually lose; it will be impossible to relax and recuperate when we most need to; and both our sex lives and our personal relationships will become atrophied.

Until we can achieve this basic priority the immediate need is for time and space. Your first and most difficult task may be to create them. Time can be found, since much of what we spend time on is not essential, whereas health and survival are. Examine your priorities, particularly the time you are expected to devote to routine and the needs of others. Take that time back; it is yours, and you need it. Space may be more difficult, particularly in family situations. Perhaps you should consider adapting your bedroom for other uses (most bedroom space is underused); forget the glamor, or remove the squalor and use the space practically. With time and space at your command you can begin to deal with stress.

The rest of this chapter is devoted to specific recommendations which will help you to recuperate and avoid exhaustion. Follow these strategies in conjunction with the activity and diet recommendations in chapters 17 and 18.

16.4 THE NEED FOR RELAXATION

Your body cannot recuperate properly if you cannot relax. The following sections offer approaches to relaxation which will be useful whatever your condition. The first deals with ways of breathing which you can adopt whenever the need arises. Then we consider strategies suitable for unwinding and preparing for sleep. Finally we discuss meditation, yoga and muscle relaxation techniques. If you can develop your own method of achieving the same objective, do so. Developing your own resources will increase your capacity to cope with stress, and this is an important part of being a competent, independent and healthy person.

16.5 BREATHING

Because breathing is automatic we take it for granted and overlook the benefits which can be gained from exerting control over it occasionally. Try this simple test—it will tell you if your normal breathing is adequate and if you are habitually slouching:

Stand with your back against a wall or door. Get as straight and upright as you can without effort, but make sure your shoulders are pushed back. Now breathe in slowly so that your chest rises; fill it as much as you can. Hold it full while you count up to four, then breathe out and let your chest fall, but keep your shoulders back. Do this five times, slowly and regularly.

Do not be alarmed if your heart starts to thump away; this is mainly relief at the pressure your change in posture has taken off it and the effect of the extra oxygen taken in through deep breathing. You may also feel a little weak or dizzy; this is another effect of unaccustomed amounts of oxygen. If you experience either or both of these effects, then in your everyday life you need to straighten up, get your shoulders back and breathe more efficiently. Go through the routine three or four times a day, and work at breathing like that *all the time*.

You probably noticed that when you stepped away from the wall you felt calmer, a little more relaxed, clearer-headed and better able to face the world. Use the routine whenever you need that little boost, breathing slower and deeper as you get more used to it.

16.6 RELAXATION METHODS

Most night schools and many health and fitness clubs offer relaxation sessions. They also offer the advantage of social contact and a change of routine. If this appeals to you, go and talk to the instructor about your needs to see if his particular class can help you. Make sure the class includes things you can do on your own at home; relaxation that depends on special equipment or circumstances is not the answer.

The next two sections describe methods you can apply on your own. The first is useful before going to bed, the second for unwinding.

16.7 PREPARING FOR SLEEP

Lie on a firm bed or soft floor in a quiet, warm, softly lit room. Make sure you are not wearing tight clothes or anything which will distract you. First make your body go as tense as possible; squeeze every muscle and make yourself rigid. Hold your breath and count to two; then, breathing slowly and deeply, make all your muscles go limp like very runny jelly. As you change from rigid to jelly, bring into your mind's eye the picture of a single object—an apple, a blue triangle, anything you can visualize easily—and concentrate totally on it for a few minutes. Imagine you are lying on a warm beach, or in a flower-filled meadow, anywhere you would like—be there! If you cannot get the initial visualization, it is usually because some part of you is still tense. See if you can locate the tense muscles, then start again and make sure they relax first. You will soon get the knack. Repeat every day and you will find that you will soon learn to relax totally. But beware—you may fall asleep when doing this exercise!

16.8 UNWINDING

First, shut the door and make sure you are not disturbed. Do the basic breathing described in section 16.5 to set you up. Put on some soft and appealing music, or if this is not possible, sing or play some music in your head, or recite poetry to yourself or just think nice thoughts. Make sure you are not wearing tight clothes or anything which distracts.

Stand loosely, close your eyes if you like, and just start to move slowly and gently; start by swaying, then move your arms slowly and loosely, and listen to the rhythm of the music or the words in your head. Listen also to what your body is telling you; locate bits that do not want to move, that are stiff and tight, and persuade them to loosen. If you have to lie down to loosen your legs and back, that is fine—do whatever you want. Forget what you may look like; just concentrate on feeling loose and good. Get the right sort of self-consciousness! After a while you may find that exuberance takes over, that you want heavy rock rather than soft and sweet music. Do not resist the urge—go with it. The dance recommendations in section 17.4 will get you started if you are not used to this sort of thing.

16.9 MEDITATION

This is one method that has proved very effective for stress management. Meditation in the classical sense does need a sympathetic teacher, but you may be able to achieve similar results by other means.

Any hobby which takes you out of the everyday rut might have a similar effect, but do not go for anything competitive or with a goal to achieve. Try keeping tropical fish and spending time just watching them. (Do not sit and watch TV; it is not the same.) Or listen to all that music you have meant to follow up on for years; work your way through Beethoven, perhaps, or learn to play something yourself—but do not rush it.

16.10 YOGA

This ancient system covers all the areas we have dealt with above. Through it you can learn appropriate methods of breathing, movement and meditation. It can be learned from books but you will make better progress if you find an appropriate course with an experienced teacher. Your local adult education center, health store or library will be able to help you find one.

There are many forms of yoga breathing exercises which can be ideal for anxiety reduction, and the stretching and relaxation exercises will help in dealing with muscular tension. Yoga can be one of the most valuable alternatives to drugs; adepts can alter the course of a great many health problems through the control they gain over their mental and physical systems.

16.11   MUSCLE RELAXATION

Some chronically anxious people find that deep-breathing exercises add to tension and make them more edgy. If this is your problem, try the following routine for deep muscle relaxation. You will need to practice regularly, ideally at least twice a day to begin with. With practice you will be able to hit the "off" switch and relax all your muscles at once. You should then be able to clear your mind and shed your anxiety (see section 16.13 for advice).

Make sure you are not disturbed. Lie on your back on a carpeted floor and work through this sequence (it may help to tape record it to avoid having to read each step):

1. With your arms lying at your side, make a tight fist and tense the muscles of your right arm. Feel them from your fist up to your shoulder. Let the tension build while you count up to five. Then relax suddenly, let your fingers fly open and spend thirty seconds feeling the relaxation from fingertips to shoulder.
2. Now, staying with your right arm, tense your fist, bend your arm at the elbow and concentrate on building tension in your upper arm. Let the tension build while you count to five (relax instantly if you feel cramp coming on), then relax as before, with your arm loose by your side, for another thirty seconds.
    Repeat 1 and 2 with the left arm.
3. Tense the muscles of your neck by lifting your head so that your chin goes onto your chest. Build the tension in your neck muscles for a count of five, and then relax for thirty seconds.
4. Tense the muscles of your face. Clamp your jaw tightly shut and pull your mouth into a grimace. Squeeze your eyes tightly shut and wrinkle your nose. Raise your eyebrows and wrinkle your forehead. See if you can manage all that at once, then relax.

5. Tense the muscles of your shoulders, chest and back. Take a deep breath, pull your shoulders back and together as if standing to attention and count up to four. Then relax and breathe out.

6. Tense the muscles of the abdomen by almost pulling your straight legs off the floor. Take a deep breath and bear down with your stomach muscles so that the pressure tends to flatten your stomach. Count to four, then relax.

7. With your legs straight and slightly apart, tense the muscles of your right buttock, then your right thigh, pushing the back of your knee to the floor as you do so, and finally tense your calf and foot. As the tension spreads down your leg, curl your foot upward so that your big toe points toward your head. (Relax immediately if you experience cramp.) Breathe in and count up to five, then relax and breathe out.

   Repeat with your left leg.

8. When you have completed this sequence take a deep breath, count up to four and then relax deeply as you breathe out. Enhance your relaxed state with slow, rhythmic deep breathing. You may feel dreamy or slightly exhilarated; use the time to explore the feelings which tensing and relaxing your muscles produced in your mind; explore the control circuits so that you can locate them with greater ease. Then count backward from five down to one, sit up, get up, and move slowly until you are fully alert once more. You will be feeling much better.

16.12 BREATHING FOR PANIC ATTACKS

A frightening aspect of panic attacks is the sensation of struggling for breath; this makes the heart thump and can cause chest pain.

You can check whether overbreathing—hyperventilation—is the cause of your problem with this simple test: First equip yourself with a paper bag; an ordinary grocery bag around six by nine inches is fine. Then sit in a comfortable chair with a clock or watch. Practice breathing at a rate of thirty to forty deep breaths per minute. This is roughly twice the normal rate of breathing, so you will have to work at it!

When you are familiar with this rate of breathing, do it continuously for five minutes. You can expect to feel light-headed and tired, and your mouth will probably go dry. Are you also starting to experience the symptoms you suffer during an anxiety attack? If so, hold the paper bag loosely over your mouth and nose and use it to rebreathe the air you exhale at your normal rate. After a short period of breathing the air from the bag, your symptoms will disappear.

If this test brought on your symptoms, you now know how to get rid of them. Make sure you have a paper bag with you and use it whenever your symptoms start. If for any reason this is not possible, when symptoms such as palpitations start, try simply holding your breath for as long as you can between breathing in and out. Develop a sustainable rhythm: in—hold—out—hold—in—hold—out— and so on.

You may think it odd that the solution to the feeling that you cannot get enough air should be actually to restrict your breathing, but you will find that it works. Overbreathing sufferers in fact breathe too often, but too shallowly. This is a common response to anxiety, though sufferers often do not recognize the cause. The danger of shallow breathing is that it upsets the chemical balance of the blood, and it can put considerable strain on the heart. Sufferers should practice the breathing strategy outlined in section 16.5. When you feel short of breath remember that you need to use each breath more fully, not breathe more often. Yoga (section 16.10) may also prove useful.

16.13 DEALING WITH WORRY

Life is full of problems and we cope with most of them, one way or another, without too much trouble. However, when particular problems become fixed and we feel we cannot deal with them, they can cause stress which becomes chronic and leads to illness.

Difficulties of this kind are a very individual matter; something which one person sees as an intractable problem will not affect another. For example, being unable to find a job makes some people ill, destroying their self-image and confidence and upsetting their relationships. Others may find it quite easy to adapt to and turn to their advantage.

Whatever the problem, it needs to be confronted. If you cannot face it alone, do so with others. But make sure you seek help from the right quarter; one reason why so many people end up on drugs is that they turn to their doctors, who may be sympathetic but have no answers to social or economic problems.

Even if you are to share your problem with someone else, you will still need to be clear in your own mind what it is that you need help with. One feature of life is that problems rarely come alone; start by writing a list of the things which are really worrying you. Take your time and think about them as objectively as you can. You may find you can cross off some things you write down either because they are not really problems or because they are not what is really troubling you. Soon you will have a few lines which are a statement of the real problems and of your feelings on their importance—a list of priorities.

Now you must make plans to deal with them, starting from the top. Whether it is your job, your relationship, your housing or something more personal and immediate, consider all the possibilities, all the sources of solutions, and work out a plan of campaign, no matter how long-term. Doing this will *in itself* be a major part of the answer, as it will give you confidence to take the next step.

16.14 CONFIDENCE

Confidence is essential for solving any problem. As with physical capacity, once you begin to use what you have, you will find that your confidence grows. Anxiety and the problems which induce it can reduce your confidence to the point where you feel trapped. The fact that you are reading this book is a sure sign that you are not at this point now, but when you next are (and it happens to all of us at times) you will need something other than drugs to get you up and away once more.

Some people find music helpful when they feel lacking in confidence—a rousing classic, perhaps, or some high-energy rock. Others find words useful—Shakespeare or a fragment of poetry that sticks in the mind. It does not matter what it is as long as it inspires you to take the next step. Do *not* use negative forces such as anger, envy or jealousy to lift you; they may work, but at the cost of more stress—the very thing which you are trying to avoid. As Duke Ellington used to put it, "let nothing disturb your beautiful personality."

Once you are up, build on it. Try some of the breathing and activity routines suggested in this and the next chapter. Activity changes your brain chemistry naturally, and that will help you. You will find you have initiated a positive cycle—so keep it going!

16.15 COUNSELING

Counseling can be very helpful with many problems, and for some it is the only answer. There are many agencies which exist solely to help with personal problems, and they are as near as your nearest phone book. A list of the larger national agencies is given at the end of this book in Appendix B, together with notes on the help they offer. Whatever your problem, and no matter how isolated you feel with it, do not hesitate to contact them if you need help. Your problem may seem overwhelming and insuperable and possibly very embarrassing to you, but they will have had a lot of experience of it; you will not be the first or the only one, so do not let the walls of your trap inhibit you. If you need help, ask for it.

One area where professional help is often the only answer is in relationship and sexual problems. Relationships tend to get locked into self-reinforcing patterns, and friends and relatives only add from one side or the other to the unsatisfactory nature of these patterns. Whatever you may believe, there are few "rights" or "wrongs" in such situations, just a lot of unhappiness that needs uninvolved but sympathetic help. Try it; you have nothing to lose and a lot to gain.

16.16 WIDER CAUSES OF STRESS

It may have occurred to you to ask, if everything is getting better (as we are led to believe), if human effort and progress are good, why are so many of us in such a state?

While we can act to deal with our individual and local problems, collectively we are doing too little to correct the forces which structure life in a way that makes stress inevitable. "Think globally, act locally" is a catchphrase used by conservationists and those concerned with our environment to help put their arguments into context. It also applies to the universal problem of stress; we need to think in global terms to understand the problem of stress and stress-related disease.

The principal generator of stress in the world is human numbers. You may not think the population explosion, and all the clichés associated with it, applies to you, but it does. While the basic needs of people cannot be met, and a higher proportion of the world's population is deprived every year, there will be pressure for resources which cannot be avoided. Techno-fixes, economic juggling, charity or any other such answers evade the basic problem: there are too many people in the global community. Until this problem is solved, all others will remain, from the possibility of nuclear holocaust to the emergence of virulent new global infections.

Human numbers are stressing every other system to its limits. Until we deal with the global cause we will remain victims of the forces we generate.

17

Activity

Human beings are designed to be very active animals. We cannot deny this basic fact. Our bodies are covered in muscle that depends upon regular use to grow and function at its best. Well-developed muscle gives our bodies a shape that we recognize as desirable and healthy. The most important muscle in the body is the heart, and like all other muscles it can be strengthened and developed to last a long time or allowed to wither and fail.

Healthy muscles give the whole body tone and resilience. Muscles act as primary energy stores; keeping them in shape keeps the blood vessels which supply the energy in good condition, and this is very beneficial for the heart.

Other systems of the body also benefit from muscular activity. The muscles which control all our activities, from breathing to excretion, are stimulated by exertion and the increased activity of the cardiovascular system. The liver, too, is stimulated by demand from the muscles, and keeping the liver in good condition is essential for health since it metabolizes all unwanted substances, from toxins to the debris of infections.

Activity also affects more subtle and apparently unconnected bodily systems. It can lift depression by causing changes in brain chemistry which alter moods, and the increased availability of oxygen makes us more alert and perceptive; the brain consumes a lot of oxygen for mental activity. When we are active, all our systems work faster and better, protecting us from common problems such as indigestion and constipation along the way.

In a word, activity is essential for a healthy life.

It seems strange that we should have to remind ourselves of this fact. We enjoy physical activity. It brings confirmation of ability and a sense of power and well-being that feels good. It keeps us youthful and enhances our looks. The problem is that most of us are conditioned to be physically inactive. Our prejudices against physical activity are deeply engrained; they began when men first began employing others to do their work for them. Since that time the idle rich have been envied by the laboring poor, and our scale of social values, of what is inferior or superior, has reinforced the acceptability of physical idleness. Technology provided another dimension: brain-workers, segregated in offices, adopted a disastrously sedentary life-style.

In education the development of our children is biased toward brain as opposed to what is derogated as brawn. And such is the way we live that the moment children cease to be lovely little things and become overactive nuisances, the universal reaction is to encourage in them an unnatural passivity. This passivity affects their attitudes toward health as well as toward life in general. Parents who themselves have been raised as passive victims raise children who perpetuate the same attitudes—attitudes of dependence on other people or on drugs, and of helplessness in the face of avoidable illness. There are few innocent bystanders in health; you are either passive, and a potential victim, or active and effective in your own cause.

SECTION INDEX

17.1　*Adapting to change*

17.2　*Start from where you are*

17.3　*Acceptable levels of activity*

17.4   *Dancing*
17.5   *Walking*
17.6   *Fitness exercises*
17.7   *Running*
17.8   *Activity for stamina*
17.9   *Activity for building and shaping*
17.10 *Some pitfalls*

17.1   ADAPTING TO CHANGE

Our bodies are marvelously adaptive, but if we live without using our physical capacity we will lose it. Years of driving to the office, working nine to five at a desk, driving home to supper, TV and bed produces the spindly, atrophied legs (and atrophied hearts) which can be seen on any beach. Eating or drinking too much adds the flabby gut, while stress adds the lined face and bellicose outlook—perfect adaptation to an unhealthy way of life and a premature death. Yet it can all be avoided; no matter how far down that road you are, it is rarely too late to turn back, and once you have done so your progress toward health will accelerate. The more your body adapts, the more you will be able to do.

Activity is the only way to increase the front-slope capacity discussed in the last chapter, and it will increase your stamina, strength and suppleness—the three S's of physical fitness. Having said that, we must now give an important warning: whatever your objective, *do NOT undertake any course of activity until you have given absolute priority to dealing with your stress level* as recommended in the previous chapter. The priorities are *relaxation, rest* and *recuperation*. Unless you achieve these, activity could add to your stress, not help reduce it. When stress levels have been reduced, physical activity can be used to increase capacity and lower them further.

17.2   START FROM WHERE YOU ARE

Ideally we should maintain a balanced mixture of mental and physical activity in our lives. We should have skills in both spheres, which would enhance our options for expression and satisfaction. Unfortunately, life tends to push us behind desks or into mindless, repetitive tasks, or leaves us isolated with a minimal role or function.

In this context exercises and other activities designed to have specific effects must be seen for what they are: compensations for a way of life which is usually far from ideal. Because such activities are a substitute, we have to be conscientious in their application and take care to ensure that they achieve the intended results.

Since we are not educated for an ideal life, and may as a consequence not be in the best physical condition, it is important to be as realistic as possible about our abilities. Most damage is done when people who are past their best suddenly decide to do something strenuous. Usually they are under the illusion that their prowess is undiminished by the years which have slipped away, and they do something to impress the children or a young lady, or in response to a challenge from a younger person. The results are entirely predictable, often painful and sometimes tragic.

We all have to start from where we are. At first you should not undertake more than *half* the amount of activity you believe you are capable of coping with. You will feel the effects for up to forty-eight hours afterward, so make sure you allow enough time for recovery. Gradually increase your activity as your capacity increases; otherwise you will be fighting yourself in an effort to recover from your excesses. "Little but often" is the best strategy; one big bash every now and then is almost a complete waste of time and effort.

You do not have to get up at dawn (unless you want to) or exercise at any specific time of the day. Nor should age prevent you from beginning, though older people should take things more slowly than the young; you also need to bear in mind that the older you are the more time you may have to devote to a gentler regime to achieve the same results.

You can in fact approach an ideal level of activity without deviating too far from your normal routine. For people who use cars for short journeys, it is all too easy to slip behind the wheel and into a coronary. Why not be a little more adventurous? Try getting on a bike, or walking. A rough rule of thumb we recommend for routine daily mobility is this: for distances of up to two or three miles, walk;

for two to five miles (more in nice weather!), use a bike; for five miles and over use public transportation; use the car only when there is no other option.

17.3 ACCEPTABLE LEVELS OF ACTIVITY

Because of individual variability it is possible to give only very rough indications. You should make your own assessment as to whether your level is adequate. Are you physically competent? Could you run half a mile to get out of trouble (or act appropriately in other emergency situations)? Could you jump out of an aircraft? Can you swim? If so, how far? Are you strong enough to be self-sufficient physically? You must decide what parameters of competence are appropriate to your life-style.

Here is a rough guide to a healthy level of activity. You should walk a brisk couple of miles every day—not stop-and-start shopping or a casual stroll, but two miles in under thirty minutes. Twice a week you should undertake some form of strenuous activity which makes you sweat for at least twenty minutes. This will cause your liver to discharge its glycogen energy stores; its subsequent recharging from fat stores and food will improve your metabolism and increase your resistance to infections. This level of activity is also necessary to have a positive affect on your cardiovascular system. But you have to be fit to undertake this much activity. The following sections give a gradual buildup to the point where you will be fit enough to improve your health.

17.4 DANCING

Anyone, even if confined to bed, can undertake some form of rhythmic movement to music. Dancing is one of the oldest forms of human recreation. It gives us self-expression, relaxation, stimulation, transcendence, communication and emotional satisfaction. Unfortunately our mundane world limits this advantageous activity mainly to the young. This is wrong; all ages need to regain the innate advantages of dance. Do not believe you are too old, too fat, too awkward or too anything else. None of that is important. You may be self-conscious—most of us are; getting into dance can turn that into something valuable: consciousness of yourself.

Dance can regenerate the very core of your being. Because it is a self-directed activity it will involve many levels of your being, both physical and mental, and create feedback loops which can build up sensations and energy that are at times almost frighteningly exhilarating; at other times dance can be just a gentle exploration of parts of yourself. In any case, the rhythms will help you unlock and grow.

Forget the rigid formulas of specific dances. What you want is spontaneous movement generated by good feelings between your body and your mind. It doesn't matter what you actually do, as long as you enjoy it and do enough of it to warm you up. Choose music which matches your mood, and let movement slide into you, slowly at first, until you become less inhibited. Your movement should pervade and persuade you and carry you along. Don't be afraid to let go; let it take you wherever it will! It may be a soft sensuous experience, or a driving physical expression of feeling, depending on your mood and needs. The important thing is to move as much of your body as you can and enjoy it. Dance as long and as often as you like, alone or in company. See if you can get your partner to join in sometimes—but remember, you are dancing for yourself.

17.5 WALKING

This most basic and healthy activity has almost become a forgotten art. Even in major cities, supposedly characterized by hustle and hurry, people slouch along at a lethargic pace.

In the absence of any other physical activity it is advisable for all ages to walk briskly—in excess of four miles an hour—for half an hour every day. For many people this single change in life-style will produce a vast improvement in health and well-being. When you do it is not important; you might be able to walk to and from work, or spend half your lunch hour walking, or leave the car (or get off the bus) a mile away from work or home and complete the journey on foot. Alternatively, make an event of it in the evening; explore your neighborhood or check out new places.

Whenever you walk, wear flat comfortable shoes—good-quality running shoes are excellent, unless you are going over rough wet ground—and suitable clothes. Get a shoulder bag or knapsack to carry a raincoat and perhaps a scarf and gloves as well; it will be essential if you get the "walking bug" and become really adventurous.

Once you are feeling the benefits of daily half-hour walks, you should consider extended walks on the weekends. Try a three- or four-hour expedition, for example, to a restaurant for lunch and back again, or around some local beauty spots. Aim for a walk that will physically tire you; get equipped and go in all weather; come home to a favorite meal and a hot bath. Make your walk an enjoyable physical activity.

On walking technique: think of the ramrod swing and stamp of the regimental sergeant-major. He looks a little comical because he exaggerates the required movements in the hope that those he is instructing pick up something of the right idea. You need not go that far, particularly if you have been doing your breathing and posture routine (see section 16.5). When you step forward, swing your leg and dig your heel in to pull you forward, push off with the ball of your foot and take longer strides than you usually would. Get the most out of each leg movement. You will find you swing your arms in order to balance the pull and push of your legs. Keep your body loose, with shoulders straight but relaxed, and breathe deeply and easily. Experience the feeling of pride that a loping stride and upright body can give you. In a matter of weeks you will find yourself striding along on healthier legs (in better shape, too), and you will be amazed at the lack of ability of those around you. When you get to this stage it may be time to move on, but don't hurry. Take your time and build up your capacity.

Vary your pace as you go; a change of pace might be better than a rest. You will feel your muscles working through a full and growing range of movements. Walk fast enough to sweat. It is good for you. It shows that your systems are working properly and it refreshes the skin.

Do not put up with pain, however. Minor muscular aches that fade with a brief rest can be ignored, but not persistent sharp pain. It is a warning that some part of your body is overloaded. Ease up, go home, rest and recover. There will be other days. Your systems are bound to be out of balance and may run out of steam for no apparent reason; perhaps they are preoccupied with fighting an infection. Next time take it a little easier and increase the pace later in your walk. Remember you are aiming to build your bodily capacity, not do a demolition job.

Above all, do not give up! Walking is an activity to continue with till you are well past ninety.

Contact the following groups for encouragement, information and company:

Walking Association, P.O. Box 37228, Tucson, AZ 85740. (602) 742-9584.
Walkways Center, 733 15th St., Suite 427, Washington, DC 20005. (202) 737-9555.
Society of Saunterers, 2461 Whitehouse Trail, Gaylord, MI 49735. (517) 732-2547.

17.6   FITNESS EXERCISES

If you are walking well and easily for half an hour each day, you may benefit from an all-around system of fitness activity. We are not going to give you one of our own since there is an excellent system ready-made. You will find it in *Physical Fitness*, a system developed by the Royal Canadian Air Force and available in two volumes, the *5BX Plan* for men and the *XBX Plan* for women. It has many advantages: the programs are graduated to suit a wide range of abilities; they take only around fifteen minutes per day; and the system may be all you need to keep perfectly fit.

17.7   RUNNING

Regular running is particularly helpful for the following conditions: cardiovascular and circulation problems, high blood pressure, liver conditions, weight loss, depression, chronic pain, premenstrual syn-drome and menstrual problems. It will also help you maintain perfect skin.

You must judge for yourself when you are ready to take up running. If you are not sufficiently fit, work your way through the preceding sections. The RCAF exercises (section 17.6) will not only get you fit, but they also make a good warm-up routine before you set off.

How much, or how little, should you run? To affect most of the conditions noted above, three or four miles two or three times a week should be quite enough. But individual variability must be taken into account; if you are small and skinny you will be able to run further than if you are tall and large. The best approach is to remember what you are trying to achieve. The key to healthy running is to do enough to persuade your liver to discharge its glycogen stores. You will be able to feel when this is happening, although you might get a little pain from your liver (just below your ribs on your right-hand side) as it registers the seriousness of your demand. "Second wind" is the com-mon description of the effect you are after, when energy suddenly flows and all the minor feelings which were inhibiting you are sud-denly replaced by exhilaration. Once this happens you should con-tinue running to burn off the energy your liver is pouring out; when you feel it running out, start to ease off. Ideally you should get back or finish your last lap at a very slow, loose jog, gently running your systems down. When your breathing and heartbeat are back near normal, stretch your arms and legs out straight several times and touch your toes as in the RCAF routine until any stiffness has gone. Then bathe or shower and relax!

As you become more fit it will take more effort to achieve this effect. You can do this either by running further or by running faster. If you opt for running faster make sure you are warmed up before you put much effort into speed. Hamstrings and joints will suffer if you do not.

Women who wish to cure hormone problems, menstrual pains and premenstrual tension will find it helpful to run at a steady rate for around half an hour (about two to three miles) each day. This will also be enough to reduce superficial fat; the further and faster you go, the more you will lose. Running this distance regularly will affect your periods; if you run four to five miles each day they may cease altogether. This is not a permanent effect; they will return once your activity level drops.

As with walking, when running regularly you should vary your stride, your pace and if possible your terrain. Plodding along the same roads can become monotonous. However, do not run along roads with much traffic; sucking in hydrocarbon exhaust is not good for you. (See also the notes on plateauing in section 17.10.)

17.8   ACTIVITY FOR STAMINA

Men who have been at risk from any form of heart disease should aim to build up stamina. It will do women no harm either. The activities noted above will do this if you put enough work in, but they can become uninteresting. Once you are fit enough to run regularly you should consider adding regular sport to your activity; perhaps this is the opportunity (or excuse) to go back to something you enjoyed in earlier years, or to try something new. Choose a sport you think you will enjoy, and try some others even if you were no good at them the last time you tried; you may be in for a pleasant surprise now that you are fitter. The following activities will build your stamina if you apply yourself to them energetically: badminton, canoeing, cycling, disco dancing (the more frenetic variety), football, gardening, gymnastics, hill walking (try backpacking for weekends on some long-distance trails), judo, running, soccer, squash, swimming and tennis.

Stamina building and cardiovascular conditioning require activity which fires up your systems so that your heart beats hard and your breathing is deep. Do not try to keep your mouth shut, but breathe the easiest and most natural way. Aim for a heart rate that does not rise above the upper limit for your age given on page 293. If you have any difficulty finding your pulse at your wrist, put your hand on your heart (at the bottom of your ribs on your left-hand side). Use a watch to get to know what your limit feels like in terms of your activity level.

WARNING: Use these figures as a guide only. Respond to your feelings and do not force your heart rate up if your body tells you it does not want to go.

DESIRABLE MAXIMUM PULSE RATE

Age	Beats per minute	Beats per 15 seconds
20–29	140	35
30–39	132	33
40–49	122	31
50–59	114	28
60–69	106	26

17.9 ACTIVITY FOR BUILDING AND SHAPING

Adding bulk or removing it from specific areas of your body can be achieved by fairly localized activity; you can develop shapely calves or bulging biceps without changing too much else, although the stimulation to hormones and adjacent muscles will tend to spread the benefits.

To increase bulk you need to concentrate on slow movements with high resistance and a low number of movement repetitions. If you wish to reduce bulk or refine shape, you need faster movements, lower resistance and a higher number of repetitions. Weight training is the ideal solution for both aims because it can be directed at the specific muscle groups you wish to develop. Make sure you warm up completely first, and combine weight training with your other activities; do not try to use it as a substitute or a short cut.

It is a good idea to join a weight-training club with an experienced staff. They will be sympathetic to your needs and usually helpful, but do beware of the oversell; commercial clubs have a variety of facilities and a range of course options, so make sure you are getting what you want and not a lot of attractive but useless extras.

Once you are fit enough to benefit from weight training, you can have exactly the sort of body you want—within certain limits. If you are short it will not make you tall, and if you have a light build there will be a limit to how bulky you can become. By the time you come to consider this option you should have a fairly realistic view of your potential.

17.10   SOME PITFALLS

Before you leave this chapter there are some things to watch out for if you are to get the maximum benefit from activity.

(a) Plateauing

This is a common problem. When you have reached a certain level of activity and fitness, your body adapts and you settle onto a stable plateau. Your regular activity becomes absorbed into your normal routine and further benefit becomes elusive.

The RCAF system (see section 17.6) avoids this problem because it is graduated and progressive. If you are not using this system you will have to vary your type of activity in order to keep your body guessing. Avoid settling into a rut; once you have achieved your initial objectives, try something different and develop as wide a mix of activities as possible. Do things that emphasize one of the S's—strength, stamina or suppleness—that you are not so good at.

(b) Obsession

Unless you wish to specialize in some sport or activity, be careful not to become obsessive about a particular routine or activity. Obsessive exercisers are akin to anorexics; both override their body responses in pursuit of some ideal which is totally illusory. Running in spite of pain or illness, or overusing the legs, can lead to lasting damage. Never use exercise to punish yourself or to demonstrate your strength of will. One aspect of this problem has to do with our internal drug systems, since the brain produces a range of substances during activity which make us feel good both during and after. This reward system that nature has devised can become addictive on its own account; as long as we get that surge of beta-endorphins, the purpose of activity can get overlooked.

(c) Self-delusion

A survey in Britain showed that many people questioned believed not only that they ought to be active for the sake of their health but also that they actually were being active. Many of them gave walking and swimming as the activities they pursued, but investigation revealed that few regularly did the things they said they did. Most of it was in their mind. This phenomenon is also observable when a particular sport is prominent on TV; when Wimbledon is on, for example, many people *say* they play tennis, and although some will be encouraged actually to do so, many will just *think* they do.

It is very easy to delude yourself into thinking that you are doing things when in fact you are not, particularly common things like walking. It is also easy, once you start an activity, to think you do it more often than is actually the case. We might say that we go running "three times a week"; some weeks this might be true, but some weeks might be missed completely. You have to be conscientious about your exercise if you want it to have the effect you desire.

(d) Rundown

Lastly, a long-term consideration. If you have spent a number of years building up to and maintaining a level of regular activity, do not suddenly stop. A moment's thought will tell you that an instant stop is as illogical as an instant start. If you have to give up, or you feel yourself losing the vigor of early years, wind down gradually. This way you will keep your systems in balance and working at the appropriate level for your age and condition.

18

Nutrition

Since eating and drinking are basic to life, since enormous effort is devoted to the science of nutrition, and since the industry which supplies most of our food is highly favored by subsidy and profit, the casual observer might imagine that we would have solved any problems that might have existed in this area of life long ago. In fact the opposite is nearer the truth. Most people in the West do not eat enough nutritious food and are deficient in vitamins and minerals. Dieting is one cause; not only does it distort the metabolism but it also distorts people's whole perception of food. Another cause is that most of the food on sale in the average store is highly suspect if not downright harmful. It would take only a small supermarket basket to collect those items which are above suspicion.

Over the last forty years there has been a revolution in the food industry. Wholesome traditional produce has been replaced by factory-farmed and processed products which have little connection with nature beyond the folksy picture printed on the pack to entice the consumer. It has taken a long time for us to acknowl-

edge that the mere fact that a product is on sale does not mean that it is good for us or even safe. Recent concern over food additives only scratches the surface of the problem. Ordinary food contains a wide variety of pesticide and drug residues—pesticides from the almost continuous crop dusting which is practiced by many farmers, and drug residues from the hormones and antibiotics fed to livestock. Even fish from the sea bring with them the residues of pesticides sprayed long ago onto the land.

We are at the top of a food chain in which artificial chemicals increase in concentration at each level from bacteria upward. It is no exaggeration to say that much of the chronic disease and general malaise which affect us, together with our increasing susceptibility to allergies, cancers and infections, can be traced back to this pollution.

The sources of most of the chemicals used to grow, process and preserve our food are the same multinational companies who manufacture the drugs which caused your concern in the first place, so in pursuing an alternative you have now come full circle. Many chemical companies have been buying agricultural seed companies in order to ensure that the seeds the farmers buy are plant strains which need artificial fertilizers and pesticides to thrive—addicted plants, if you like. They also manufacture all the veterinary drugs used in intensive farming. There is not one level of the food-supply chain that does not bear the fingerprints of the chemical industry: fumigants and antifungals for storing the harvest, growth-inhibiting hormones to prevent plants from sprouting, colorings and preservatives to keep food looking fresh, hydrolizers and antioxidants to prolong shelf life—the list is endless. A significant proportion of the 35,000 artificial chemicals now in common use is introduced by the food industry somewhere along the line from field to table. There are around 3,500 different additives and around 3,000 different colorings in use. Even the paper bag you buy food in is likely to be as much plastic as wood pulp.

It may be true that each of the substances involved in modern food production is safe in low concentrations for the majority of people, and that many people will be able to cope for some time on a diet which contains many such substances; but it is only the very fortunate who have bodies efficient enough to cope day after day with the assault the modern food industry delivers. The fact is that as this assault grows in intensity and complexity, fewer people are able to cope with it. Our bodies are forced to work harder as each new molecule has to be assessed and dealt with by protective systems which are finely tuned to deal with a range of substances encountered during our evolution. This evolution was relatively slow; now we simply cannot keep up with what is happening, and breakdown is inevitable.

SECTION INDEX

18.1   *Fats*
18.2   *Organic foods*
18.3   *High-fiber foods*
18.4   *Specific nutrients*
18.5   *Amino acids*
18.6   *Foods that protect against yeast and fungal infections*
18.7   *Foods that aid female hormone balance*
18.8   *Food allergy and elimination diets*
18.9   *Foods that give you a metabolic jolt*
18.10   *Food additives*
18.11   *Sugar*
18.12   *Salt*

18.1 FATS

Over the last few decades the largest single change in our diet has been the consumption of an increasing proportion of fat. Not all fats are harmful—pure, cold-pressed vegetable oils such as olive and sunflower oil are fine—but our diet is larded with saturated and processed fats which are. Whether or not they are harmful in themselves is a matter of debate, but what is beyond doubt is that they are contaminated with drug and pesticide residues and oxidation products which are hazardous. These fats are the ones to avoid.

Today 40 percent of our food energy is derived from fats. This might strike you as odd or unlikely since in recent years many men and women have been dieting to lose weight and have been more conscious of the amount of fat they eat. Indeed, butchers complain they cannot sell fat cuts, and even hamburger has to be lean. So where is the fat coming from?

Once again we have to look at the way the food industry operates. While consumers have been rejecting fat, the food industry has been busily inventing new ways of selling it. In addition to the obvious sources such as butter, cheese and milk, all manufactured meat products are at least as high in fat as the original animal was (many are as high in bone, gristle and other parts as well). Cookies, snack cakes, snack pies and candies—all those packaged goodies—are also good ways to sell fat, as are ready-made meals, convenience foods, fast foods, snacks and anything fried. If you need to reduce your fat consumption, avoid anything processed by the food industry, and also avoid most foods derived from animal sources.

Specifically, you should use skim milk, and do not have more than a couple of ounces of low-fat cheese daily; avoid fatty cheeses such as Cheddar and cream cheese. Cut your intake of all processed and refined fats including butter, margarine, drippings, lard, sour cream and sweet cream; use cold-pressed oils such as olive and sunflower oil for cooking and salad dressings. Get out of the habit of buttering your bread; choose bread fillings that do not need butter, such as boiled eggs or mashed banana, and cut your bread thick.

Ideally, you should adopt a diet free of animal products apart from fish. The pollutants in animal fats can damage your arteries and reduce your body's ability to deal with stress hormones.

Do not try to cut all fat out of your diet, however; this would be harmful to your health. Some fats (known as essential fatty acids) are vital to protect you from a wide range of ills, from heart disease to allergies. These fats are found in unprocessed fish and plant oils, but they are damaged by processing (e.g., margarine manufacture). Be sure to eat foods that contain these beneficial fats every day. Good sources include fresh fish, especially oily varieties such as herring or sardines; nuts and seeds such as sunflower seeds; oily vegetables such as avocados; and cold-pressed plant oils, especially linseed.

18.2 ORGANIC FOODS

With so many pitfalls in achieving adequate nutrition, what can be done? Fortunately there is growing awareness of the need for radical change, and in the case of food the ideal solution is the only solution: *eat organically produced foods and filter your tap water or drink bottled mineral waters.* Excessive and impossible? Twenty years ago most people would have thought so; ten years ago you might have been thought a little cranky; today it is the only way to ensure that what you are eating and drinking is not harming you. In changing over to this regime, you will be joining a sizable minority who have already done so.

If you also adopt the traditional recommendation of dietitians—a well-balanced diet—you will have few if any of the multitude of problems which confront people on a processed and denatured diet. For most people, "well balanced" generally means more fresh fruit (washed in warm water or peeled to remove pesticide residues if not organically produced—most fruit is not) and fresh vegetables, preferably raw rather than cooked, and more nuts, seeds and grains. There are three food rules:

1. Organic is best; always go for the best. It may cost more but it is worth it.
2. Good food is food which will go bad. You should buy fresh food and eat it at its best. If it lasts a long time, it is usually because it has been treated with preservatives. The exceptions are dried beans, grains and fruits. Roots such as onions, potatoes, turnips and carrots are usually sprayed with antifungals and hormones to prevent them from sprouting in the spring as they naturally would. Organic roots are not sprayed, so you may not have continuous supplies.
3. The best food is the least processed food. You might think that fresh fruit would be minimally processed, but that isn't always the case. Orange trees, for example, are now injected with dye to avoid

unripe fruit being rejected because of green blotches, so you should be wary of out-of-season produce. Always aim for food which has had the least done to it.

Whole foods—foods which have had none of their edible parts removed—are obviously superior although they may not always be organic. For example, consider the many forms of rice sold in large supermarkets. There are various types of white and "quick-cooking" rice; these have been polished and their natural bran coating, which contains important B-group vitamins, minerals and protein, has been removed. Don't buy white rice. Brown rice, with its bran coat and a reasonable level of nutrients, is a type of whole food; organic brown rice, which is highest in nutrients, is the best and tastiest type you can get. Whole foods are generally darker in color and rougher in texture than other foods. You can't usually cook light and fluffy dishes with them, but they have far more flavor and they are what your body was designed to digest.

The best sources of organic foods are likely to be your local health-food stores. Study the label and question the staff carefully to find out whether the product is unsprayed and organically grown, because there are comparatively few stores that sell only organic food. "Health foods" are, regrettably, no more likely to be pesticide-free than any others, unless they are specifically marked as such. Some supermarkets are beginning to sell organic food; encourage them by asking for food they do not yet have on the shelves. As consumer demand grows, pure organic food will become the norm; the sooner you add your purchasing power to the demand, the better for you and everyone else.

There are some old established brands that have managed to retain their integrity. Their products may not be 100% organic but the label will state this where it is the case. Note the names, ask for their produce as often as possible and buy them as a matter of course.

Look for Erewhon Trading Company, Mountain Ark Trading Company and Autumn Harvest Natural Foods. Organic flours are available from various millers; we recommend Arrowhead Mill whole wheat flour; it makes the most delicious bread. If you have difficulty in finding organic food, write to the firms listed in Appendix B; a self-addressed envelope with your inquiry would probably be appreciated. Further information is available in the *East West Journal* (P.O. Box 1200, Brookline, MA 02147).

Remember, though, that nature is not perfect. The artificially perfect produce of the past will be replaced by imperfect but totally wholesome produce in the future. And strangely enough your best guarantee to the safety of food may be those things usually thought of as pests. If there are aphids on the lettuce, the odd caterpillar in the cabbage or a maggot in an apple, you can be fairly sure that what is safe for them is safe for you. Try looking upon these humble creatures as the modern equivalent of the miner's canary; as long as the canary sang, the miners knew they were safe from poisonous gas. Where insects are happy, you are safe; where they are being poisoned, so are you.

18.3   HIGH-FIBER FOODS

Fiber is found in all vegetables, fruits and grains but not in animal products such as meat and dairy products. A balanced organic diet will provide all the fiber you need, whereas processed food lacks not only important minerals and vitamins but also the bulk which is essential for the large intestine to function normally.

You should eat large amounts of unrefined carbohydrate foods—a high-fiber diet. This means lots of fresh vegetables, especially peas, beans, lentils, bean sprouts (preferably homegrown and raw), potatoes (boiled or baked in their skins), whole-grain bread, brown rice, whole-grain pasta and oatmeal (excellent for breakfast). You should also eat raw fruit, particularly figs, grapes, apples and pears. There should be no need to add bran (why was it removed in the first place?) or bran-based bulking agents to your diet; these reduce the uptake of trace minerals in the intestine and for that reason are not the best way of adding fiber. If you eat your food whole, with nothing taken out (and nothing put in), the fiber will be there in its most valuable and nutritious form.

If you have been eating a low-fiber, highly refined diet for some years, you may find that a sudden change to a high-fiber diet gives you gas and an uncomfortable swollen belly. Do not give up; just allow more time for the transition. Increase the quantity of fiber in your diet slowly but steadily. When the bowel does not have sufficient bulk of food on which to contract, painful disruption is much more probable. Gradually increase the fiber content of your diet by eating more high-fiber foods.

18.4 SPECIFIC NUTRIENTS

A balanced organic diet will provide all the specific nutrients most people require, but some individuals and certain conditions will benefit from increased quantities. Ideally these should be obtained from natural sources; artificial substitutes are not as good.

A word about smoking: not only does it damage respiratory membranes but it also leads to reduced levels of important vitamins. Give it up, and eat extra fresh fruit and vegetables to make up for vitamin deficiencies. Some people find that these two complimentary actions are enough to banish a host of minor ailments.

(a) Vitamin A

Vitamin A is essential for a healthy immune system, for eyesight and good skin. People who get too little vitamin A in their diet are more likely to develop cancer. The best sources of vitamin A are fresh vegetables, particularly carrots, green vegetables, peas, peppers, tomatoes and cress; ripe fruit with orange-colored flesh, especially cantaloupes, mangoes, apricots and peaches; free-range eggs; oily fish such as sardines and salmon; and organic liver.

(b) B-group vitamins

B-group vitamins are important for general well-being. They protect against stress and the effects of toxins. Rich sources are bread and other whole-grain products, wheat germ and yeast.

(c) Niacin (nicotinic acid)

Niacin is a B-group vitamin which acts with chromium (section 18.4(m)) in the body to maintain a healthy blood sugar level. It is found in whole grains but is largely lost in processing. The richest source is peanuts. It is also present in meat, poultry, fish (particularly mackerel, salmon, tuna and sardines), fresh peas and broad or fava beans.

(d) Folic acid

Folic acid, or folate, is especially important for expectant mothers. It also protects against the effects of environmental toxins. It is found in green vegetables, especially cabbage, broccoli, Brussels sprouts, peas, beans and bean sprouts, as well as in avocados, melons, free-range eggs, almonds and walnuts. Avoid irradiated food; irradiation destroys folic acid.

(e) Vitamin B$_6$

Vitamin B$_6$ (pyridoxine) is necessary to maintain the biochemical balance of the brain and is involved in carbohydrate metabolism. It is particularly plentiful in walnuts, hazelnuts, peanuts, turkey, bananas, whole grains, yeast extract, and sardines, mackerel and other oily fish. Women who suffer from depression or hormone problems should take supplements of B$_6$.

(f) Vitamin C

Vitamin C protects against damage by pathogens, toxins and environmental pollutants. It is essential for immunity to infection; your need for vitamin C will rise during infection. The richest sources of vitamin C are fruits, especially citrus and berry fruits (oranges, grapefruit, strawberries, blackberries, gooseberries, etc.), litchis, mangoes and guavas; other good sources are potatoes—especially new potatoes—green vegetables and salads.

(g) Vitamin D

Vitamin D is necessary for healthy bones. Get your vitamin D from regular exposure to sunshine, especially in winter.

(h) Vitamin E

Vitamin E promotes healing and protects your body from the ravages of time and environmental pollution. Sunflower seeds are an especially good source of vitamin E; also almonds, hazelnuts, peanuts, fish eggs, sweet potatoes, avocados and blackberries (wild are best of all).

(i) Iron

This is important for high immunity and for conditions which involve blood loss and anemia. The food richest in iron is liver, though that is also where toxic residues are concentrated, so unless you can get organically produced liver, the chemical loading could outweigh any benefits. You could buy in bulk from a reliable supplier and freeze it. Other foods rich in iron are dark meats, lentils, peas, leeks, broccoli, spring greens, watercress, radishes, parsley, and haricot, mung and butter beans. Good fruit sources are dried apricots, figs, raisins, prunes, blackberries, blueberries, raspberries and loganberries. Include as many of these in your daily diet as possible.

Boost your iron uptake by avoiding tea, coffee and soda pop; drink only water, wine or fruit juice with meals. Avoid processed foods such as reconstituted meat products and "fake" fish, mass-produced ham and frozen poultry, which may include additives that interfere with iron absorption.

(j) Zinc

Today's overprocessed diet has produced widespread zinc deficiency which results in poor resistance to infection, reduced sense of taste (so processed food may taste great to those it has robbed of the power to taste what it is *really* like) and poor skin. Zinc is often lacking in diabetics (see also section 18.4(m)). A balanced whole-food diet (see section 18.2) should supply ample quantities. Particularly rich sources are whole grains and nuts, whole-grain bread and pasta, and brown rice. Eat plenty to keep zinc levels high. Check your zinc levels with a taste test available from health-food stores to see whether you need supplements.

(k) Manganese

Manganese is necessary for the production of interferon in the body and for regulating blood sugar. High-manganese foods include almonds, hazelnuts, chestnuts, peas, avocados, whole-meal bread and oats.

(l) Magnesium

Often lacking in diabetics, heart-disease sufferers and people with kidney stones, magnesium reduces the risk of spasms in the arteries. It is found in almonds, Brazil nuts, cashews, whole-grain products, corn, spinach and bananas.

(m) Chromium

Chromium is an essential trace mineral for sugar metabolism. Brewer's yeast is very rich in chromium and beans, vegetables and whole grains also contain it. As with other trace minerals, concentrations are likely to be higher in organically grown produce. One reason for the current epidemic of diabetes could be that modern processing and production methods remove this vital mineral. Absorption from tablets is poor, so supplements are *not* the answer. A nutritionally rich organic whole-food diet (section 18.2) will supply all you need.

(n) Potassium

Potassium is important for a proper balance of salt and water in our bodies. It protects against high blood pressure and is essential for proper nerve function. It is found in fresh fruit, particularly bananas, dried fruit, grapes, cantaloupes and peaches, as well as in seeds and in vegetables. Much is lost in boiling, so eat vegetables raw or baked if possible; baked potatoes contain twice as much as boiled potatoes.

(o) Essential fatty acids

These are derived from vegetable sources and fish; they are essential for healthy metabolic functioning. Essential fatty acid deficiency is believed to be very common because modern food processing can change these substances to forms that cannot fulfill their important roles in the body. Evening primrose oil is a very rich source of these nutrients. Increase your dietary intake of essential fatty acids by supplementing your diet with wheat germ, seeds and seed oils (particularly linseed), and eating more fish. Eating hard margarine and other forms of processed vegetable fat can increase your need for essential fatty acids; soft margarine is better for you. Best of all, replace these products with tahini (sesame-seed spread) or nut butter.

18.5   AMINO ACIDS

(a) Cysteine and methionine

These are important for detoxification and good liver function. The best sources are eggs, cashew nuts, Brazil nuts, walnuts, sunflower seeds and fish.

(b) Tryptophan

Tryptophan aids sleep. Although it is present in many high-protein foods, it is selectively absorbed by the brain after meals containing carbohydrate. The easiest way to raise brain tryptophan levels is to eat a large baked potato with a sprinkling of cheese. A bowl of cereal or a sandwich will have a similar but lesser effect.

18.6   FOODS THAT PROTECT AGAINST YEAST AND FUNGAL INFECTIONS

An overgrowth of yeast (*Candida albicans,* or thrush) in the gut can produce a wide variety of symptoms. It is particularly likely to develop some weeks or occasionally months after a course of antibiotic or steroid drugs. Eat natural live yogurt three times a day, and have an avocado with a vinaigrette of two parts olive oil and one part organic cider or wine vinegar every day for two weeks. This will help rebalance the natural flora in your gut.

A diet of these foods, plus well-cooked free-range eggs, sunflower seeds and plenty of whole-grain bread, will help build and maintain your defenses against fungal infections.

18.7   FOODS THAT AID FEMALE HORMONE BALANCE

Sufferers from premenstrual syndrome should ensure that they eat enough food during the second half of their cycle. Do not skip meals, and forget about calories (read Cannon and Enzig's *Dieting Makes You Fat* instead). Eat plenty of fresh fruit, especially citrus fruit, and vegetables. PMS sufferers tend to have lower-than-average magnesium levels, so increase your intake of foods noted in section 18.4(*l*). Unprocessed oils such as olive and sunflower oil are valuable, as are nuts, seeds, avocados and fresh fish.

18.8   FOOD ALLERGY AND ELIMINATION DIETS

Food-related reactions are very controversial. Some allergists and clinical ecologists believe that adverse reactions to foods are responsible for the majority of emotional problems and for the ill-defined subclinical malaise which many people in our society suffer. A substantial body of pediatricians believes that food additives are largely responsible for hyperactivity in children. Yet many mainstream doctors still act as though sensitivity to foods and additives were very rare and unrelated to emotional, behavioral and other problems. It is true that the food-allergy bandwagon has attracted many people whose problems may have an entirely different basis, but we would be foolish to dismiss the role that chemicals in food can play in determining mood and reactions to stress. If you cannot see any other reason for an emotional problem, then you should certainly consider food allergy. Even if you know that your state is linked with some other precipitating factor, you can only improve things by eating appropriately.

Before you consider any elimination or specialized diet for allergic problems, make sure you have followed the recommendations in section 18.2. They will probably be enough to return your digestive immune system to healthy functioning. You must also recognize that allergic reactions can be highly individual, so the experience of others may not be of much use to you. If your problem persists, proceed cautiously with your exploration of it; avoid classifying whole groups of foods such as nuts or greens as the culprits; the problem is likely to be one particular nut or green vegetable, not all of them.

Allergy frequently develops to staple foods such as milk, wheat and eggs. Often the problem is with the forms of such foods which are most common in our culture: cow's milk, white flour and intensively produced eggs. These are all polluted with chemicals which are perfectly capable of setting up allergic reactions: drug residues in the milk; synthetic color in egg yolks; bleach, "improvers" and pesticide residues in the flour. A change to goat's milk, organic whole-wheat flour products and free-range eggs may be enough to overcome any problems.

Sophisticated elimination diets have been worked out for allergy sufferers, but these are not usually necessary. However, if you believe that your problem is related to foods in a more complex way than is suggested above, read *Eating Dangerously* (Harcourt Brace, 1976) by Richard Mackarness. If you suspect a particular food, try eliminating it from your diet for a couple of weeks; if this resolves the problem, you have the answer. Milk and dairy products, wheat, corn, coffee, tea and citrus fruits are common offenders. Others are fish, yeast, chocolate, nuts, pork and bacon, tea and of course food additives, preservatives and synthetic colorings (see section 18.10).

18.9 FOODS THAT GIVE YOU A METABOLIC JOLT

Many minor metabolic problems, and some more serious emotional ones, can be traced to elements of the diet. This is more probable if your diet is high in substances which can have a stimulating effect on parts of your metabolism, producing an internal imbalance which your body tends to overcorrect, thus making things worse. What these substances are will depend on the interaction between your body and what you eat; one substance may produce a strong reaction in you and no perceptible reaction in a friend.

Substances to watch out for include coffee, tea, chocolate, soft drinks, sugar, salt and synthetic food additives (see section 18.10). All of these can stimulate you temporarily, making relaxation more difficult and causing rebound depression later. Give up strong tea, coffee and cola-type drinks completely, and substitute pure fruit juice, perhaps diluted with Perrier or other bottled water. Stop eating sweets, cookies and chocolate; do not use artificial sweeteners— these are particularly bad, as they fool many body systems; avoid processed foods, especially desserts and other highly colored products. Follow the recommendations given in section 18.2.

18.10   FOOD ADDITIVES

Individuals react differently to different food additives. For some people, certain additives (especially preservatives and synthetic colors) can be dangerous allergy triggers; others may not be aware of any problems with them. We believe it is wise to avoid as many food additives as possible; good food should not need chemicals. Most additives are used primarily to make poor-quality food seem attractive; they add nothing to its nutritional value. Information is not available on flavorings; if a label indicates that artificial flavors have been added, there is no way to tell what chemicals may be used or what adverse effects they may have.

Refer to the table below for guidance.

COLORS

Beware	Suspect	Safe
FD&C yellow no. 5 (tartrazine)	Cochineal red	Turmeric
FD&C yellow no. 10 (quinoline yellow)	Aluminum	Curcumin
FD&C yellow no. 6 (orange yellow S)	Caramel	Riboflavin
Azorubine		Lactoflavin
FD&C red no. 40		Chlorophyll

Beware	Suspect	Safe
FD&C red no. 3		Carbon
Carminic acid	·	Carotenes
Patent blue		Anthocyanins
FD&C blue no. 1		Chalk
FD&C blue no. 2		Titanium oxide
FD&C green no. 3		Iron oxides
Lithol-rubin BK		
Orange B		

PRESERVATIVES

Beware	Suspect	Safe
Benzoic acid	Formic acid	Sorbic acid
Benzoates	Formates	Acetic acid
Sulfur dioxide	Lactic acid	Acetates
Sulfites and disulfites		Propionic acid
Diphenyl ketone		Propionates
Orthophenylphenol		
Sodium nitrite		
Sodium nitrate		
Potassium nitrite		

ANTIOXIDANTS, EMULSIFIERS, STABILIZERS, MISCELLANEOUS

Beware	Suspect	Safe
Gallates	Lactates	Ascorbic acid
BHA	Carrageenan	Ascorbates
BHT	Acacia gum	Tocopherols
Polyphosphates	Tartrates	Lecithins
Silicates	Phosphatides	Citric acid
	Salts of fatty acids	Citrates
	Monoglycerides	Tartaric acid
	Diglycerides	Tartrates
	Sorbitol	Alginates
		Pectin
		Cellulose

FLAVOR ENHANCERS

Beware	Safe
Glutamic acid	Beeswax
Monosodium glutamate (MSG)	Carnauba wax
Glutamates	Shellac
Inosinate	
Maltol	
Chlorine	

18.11 SUGAR

Sugar consumption has been convincingly linked with a wide range of diseases. You should avoid refined white sugar. It would be best to avoid all added sweetening. Most fruits are naturally very sweet and may be eaten instead. If you have what is commonly called "a sweet tooth," do not substitute "diet" products laced with synthetic chemicals or other artificial sweeteners; they tend to deplete your body of micronutrients as well as having other effects (see section 18.9).

If you are especially sensitive to sugar, fresh fruit should be eaten with caution; ripe fruit can be very sweet and may push your blood sugar up very quickly. Grapefruit and similar sharp fruits are not as likely to cause this problem, but you will have to learn how your body responds to each type.

Diabetics need more vitamin C than nondiabetics, so if you are not having at least a pound of fresh fruit each day (being careful of the varying carbohydrate content) you should have more of the vegetables noted in section 18.4(f).

18.12 SALT

Most people eat too much salt. It is especially bad for those with high blood pressure. The best way to cut salt consumption is to avoid processed foods and eat more raw food. Keeping your intake of fruit and vegetables high will also help to prevent salt problems; the potassium they contain will help to balance the sodium.

19

How to Join the Healthy Minority

IF you have used this book as we suggested at the beginning, you will have arrived at this point with a plan of action based on the last three chapters and a rough idea of how to build it into your life.

You will have noticed that some of our recommendations are not very specific and that there is a lot of overlap between things which are good for one condition and those which are good for others. Foods which provide one vitamin or mineral also provide others. There is no great mystery in this; being healthy is only a matter of getting a fairly small number of things right. This was summed up very well by Professor Thomas McKeown in his classic critique, *The Role of Medicine*, where he wrote,

> The determinants of health can be stated simply. Those who are fortunate enough to be born free of significant congenital disease or disability will remain well if three basic needs are met. They must be adequately fed; they must be protected from a wide range of hazards in

the environment; and they must not depart radically from the patterns of personal behaviour under which man evolved—for example by smoking, overeating, or sedentary living.

You now have the means to meet these requirements of health. Being adequately fed depends on both the quality and the quantity of what you eat. Organic whole foods, with minimally processed and additive-free substitutes on occasions, will meet all your needs provided that you eat enough of them. Women obsessed with slimming *must* eat enough if they wish to lose weight, otherwise their bodies will believe they are living in conditions of famine and will hoard fat, slow their metabolic rate and even convert healthy lean tissue into fat. You must have the confidence to forget calories and pounds and think about taste and quality instead. Men generally do not have problems eating; their problem is with *what* they eat. You know what to do about that.

Add to adequate nutrition a suitable balance in other areas of your life and you are more than halfway there. Your priorities should be to give up smoking (provided that you have replaced its support function), attend to stress levels and make sure you are always well rested. You can then add activity to build capacity, reduce weight and create more energy.

Although these factors are the same for all of us, the way in which you put them together, the emphasis you give to each and the exact diet and activity regimes you develop will be unique to you. We each have our own life dynamic which is determined by our interaction with the world we live in. There has to be a balance in this interaction, and only you can bring all these factors together in the right mix to create it.

Learning to do this, and to alter relevant factors as our lives change and we age, should be one of the principal objectives of our education system. What can be more important than to understand how to have the best chance of remaining healthy, of fulfilling our potential and enjoying the best possible life? This question raises further questions of priorities and inevitably of politics, for health in the widest sense *is* a question of politics. Not, we hasten to add, the politics that are paraded before us by the media, where questions of health are equated with sterile debates on the amount of funding given to health care. The real political questions of health which are relevant to the majority of people are rarely debated.

Let us look, for example, at the basic human need referred to above, to be protected from "a wide range of hazards in the environment." It could be argued that the original purpose of politics was to answer this need; clearly it is only by social action that large-scale hazards can be dealt with; the elimination of smallpox required global political agreement and widespread social action. In everyday terms such things as food and clothes and houses provide our basic protection, and we can all ensure that these are sufficient to maintain our health. In social terms, however, it seems as if most of our actions are having the opposite effect. Rather than improving our protection, we are every day exposing ourselves to a greater number of environmental hazards: noise, fumes, polluted food, contaminated water, environmental degradation and radioactive waste. Yet these things do not happen by chance; "they" may be doing it, but we are responsible for "them." Just as we cannot remain passive and expect medicine to pick up the pieces of our ruined health, so we cannot remain passive and expect to be able to create health in an environment which continually pushes us toward illness.

In the eighteenth century the great British social reformers understood that infectious diseases, the major killers of those days, thrived because of *social* conditions that existed at that time. Poor housing, lack of clean water, minimal sewage disposal and ignorance of hygiene and nutrition all contributed to conditions which were excellent for typhoid, smallpox, tuberculosis and other lethal pathogens. It was as a result of fundamental social reforms that these diseases began to be eradicated long before specific medical measures were developed. In the late twentieth century we require reform of even greater magnitude. Just as medicine now makes a major contribution to ill health, so our application of technological advances in hygiene and nutrition now makes us more rather than less prone to illness. Victorian sewage disposal contributed to health; our continued piping of it into the sea (along with other wastes) creates a major environmental hazard. Carbolic soap and water banished much illness arising from bad hygiene; today, in our obsession with cleanliness, our use of perfumed biological detergents, sprays, fresheners, perfumes and deodorants constitutes a major source of chemical pollution causing allergic, asthmatic and skin diseases as well as compromising our immune systems.

The reform we require is in our *culture*. The diseases which are the killers today are produced not by social deprivation but by the life-style and ethic of our Western industrialized culture. As this culture spreads around the world it takes with it heart disease, diabetes, cancer, allergies and bronchial problems. Populations which were previously free of these conditions now develop them; in adopting our way of life they also suffer our ways of death. Reform in our culture is bound to be difficult—all reforms are, because they go against the vested interest of the status quo—but it can be achieved.

You have begun the process of reform by reading this book and understanding how you may be healthy rather than a victim of illness. Cultural reform requires changing our understanding, changing the way we think, changing our basic beliefs about things in our culture. When a new understanding becomes dominant this reform will have been achieved. By acting individually and together we can create a world in which the healthy minority will have become the majority. In the long run this is the only way we will defeat our modern diseases.

If you believe that this approach is logical and worth while, join with others to influence the health of our planet; environmental groups would like your help.

APPENDIXES

Appendix A

Information About Drugs and Health Care

Organizations

American Foundation for Alternative Health Care, 25 Landfield Ave., Monticello, NY 12701. (914) 794–8181. An information and resource center for alternative health care.

Center for Medical Consumers and Health Care Information, 237 Thompson St., New York, NY 10012. (212) 674–7105. Information on drugs, health and associated matters. Excellent free-access library.

Council on Health Information and Education, 444 Lincoln Blvd., Venice, CA 90291. Disseminates information on health care.

Wellness and Health Activation Networks, P.O. Box 923, Vienna, VA 22180. (703) 281–3830.

Books

Physicians' Desk Reference (PDR). Medical Economics Company, Inc. This is the doctor's reference book about medicines; it gives detailed information on the drugs in all prescribed products, with their indications, warnings and adverse effects. New editions are published every year.

Physicians' Desk Reference (PDR) for Nonprescription Drugs. This gives detailed information about over-the-counter medicines.

Pills, Profits and Politics, by Milton Silverman and Philip Lee. University of California Press, 1976. A detailed critique of American drug use.

Appendix B

Organic Food Suppliers

Mail-order sources

Check the labels; some of these companies also market food that is not grown by organic methods.

Arrowhead Mill
P.O. Box 2059
Hereford, TX 79045

Autumn Harvest Natural Foods,
   Ltd.
1029 Davis St.
Evanston, IL 60201

Birkett Mills
P.O. Box 440 A
Penn Yan, NY 14527

Butte Creek Mill
402 Royal Ave. N
Eagle Point, OR 97524

Calloway Gardens Country Store
Highway 27
Pine Mountain, GA 31822

Erewhon Trading Company
236 Washington St.
Brookline, MA 02146
1–800–222–8028

Fangorn Organic Farm
Rte. 3, Box 141B
Rocky Mount, VA 24151

Flory Brothers
841 Flory Mill Rd.
Lancaster, PA 17601

Four Chimneys Farm Winery
Himrod-on-Seneca, NY 14842
(607) 243–7502

Great Valley Mills
Quakertown, PA 18951

Grover Co.
2111 S. Industrial Park Ave.
Temple, AZ 85282

Hodgson Mill Enterprise, Inc.
P.O. Box 126
Gainesville, MO 65655

Homestead Flour
911 W. Camden Rd.
Montgomery, MI 49255

Kenyon's Grist Mill
Usquepaugh, RI 02836

Letoba Farm Foods
Box 180, Rte. 3
Lyons, KS 67554

Mountain Ark Trading Company
Fayetteville, AR 72701
1–800–643–8909

New Hope Mills
R.R. 2
Moravia, NY 13118

Old Mill of Guilford
Box 623, Rte. 1
Oak Ridge, NC 27310

Shiloh Farms
Box 97, Highway 59
Sulphur Springs, AR 72768

Vermont Country Store
Weston, VT 05161

Walnut Acres
Penns Creek, PA 17862

Wilson Milling Co.
P.O. Box 481
La Cross, KS 67548

Retail Suppliers of Organic Foods

The stores listed offer organic produce and staples. Many mail-order items on request.

New England

Baldwin Hill Bakery
Baldwin Hill Rd. (off Rte. 2A)
Phillipston, MA 01331
(617) 249–4691

Good Day Market Cooperative
155 Brackett St.
Portland, ME 04102
(207) 772–4937

Hartman's Back to Basics
250 Main St.
East Greenwich, RI 02818
(401) 885–2679

The Whole Grocer
118 Congress St.
Eastern Promenade
Portland, ME 04101
(207) 774–7711

New York

Commodities
117 Hudson St.
New York, NY 10013
(212) 334-8330

Laughing Gull Organics
555 North Country Rd.
St. James, NY 11780
(516) 584-7363

MacDonald's Farm Market
and Natural Food Store
2 West Main St.
Trumansburg, NY 14886
(607) 387-5225

Mid-Atlantic

Earth Things, Inc.
106 Rte. 46
Rockaway, NJ 07866
(201) 627-4610

Harvestin Natural Foods
12 Locust Lane
Westminster, MD 21157

Valley Health Foods
2571 Huntingdon Pike
Huntingdon Valley, PA 19006
(215) 947-4585

The Cash Grocer, Inc.
1313 King St.
Alexandria, VA 22314
(703) 549-9544

The Grow-cery
6526 Landsdowne Ave.
Philadelphia, PA 19151
(215) 877-5902

Midwest

New City Market
1810 N. Halstead St.
Chicago, IL 60614
(312) 280-7600

The Outpost Natural Foods
Cooperative
3500 North Holton
Milwaukee, WI 53212
(414) 961-2597

Springfield Community Foods
300 N. Waverly
Springfield, MO 65802
(417) 866-1337

South

Bread of Life
Health Food Store
1575 NE 26th St.
Fort Lauderdale, FL 33305
(305) 566-2799

Natural Health Producers
5531 Richmond
Houston, TX 77056
(713) 783-8444

West

Aline's Natural Foods &
Wholesome Living Products
Alpha Beta Plaza, Farmers Lane
Santa Rosa, CA 94505
(707) 526-4912

Totality House Organic Produce
17 Fourth Ave.
Chula Vista, CA 92010
(619) 425-2813

Northwest

Whole Earth Exchange
2600 College Rd.
Box 80228
Fairbanks, AK 99708
(907) 479–2052

Canada

Baldwin Natural Foods
20½ Baldwin St.
Toronto M5T 1L2
Canada
(416) 979–1777

The Big Carrot
355 Danforth Ave.
Toronto M4K 1N7
Canada
(416) 466–2129

Appendix C

Bibliography

Adam, K., and I. Oswald. "Sleep helps healing." *British Medical Journal,* 1984.

Beller, A. S. *Fat and Thin.* Farrar, Straus & Giroux, 1977.

Blackley, C. H. *Hayfever: Its Causes, Treatment, and Effective Prevention.* Ballière, 1880.

Bland, J., ed. *Medical Applications of Clinical Nutrition.* Keats, 1983.

British Medical Association and Pharmaceutical Society of Great Britain. *British National Formulary.* The Pharmaceutical Press, 1986.

Brush, M. *Understanding Premenstrual Tension.* Pan, 1984.

Byrivers, P. *Goodbye to Arthritis.* G. K. Hall, 1986.

Cannon, G., and H. Einzig. *Dieting Makes You Fat.* Simon & Schuster, 1985.

Comfort, A. *The Joy of Sex.* Fireside, 1974.

Doll, R., and R. Peto. *The Causes of Cancer.* Oxford University Press, 1981.

Dong, D. *New Hope for Arthritics.* Granada, 1983.

Doull, J., et al., eds. *Casarett and Doull's Toxicology: The Basic Science of Poisons.* Macmillan, 1980.

Eagle, R. *A Guide to Alternative Medicine.* BBC, 1980.

Epstein, S. *The Politics of Cancer.* Sierra Club Books, 1978.

Evans, P. *Cystitis.* Beekman, 1979.

Forbes, A. *The Bristol Detox Diet for Cancer Patients*. Keats, 1985.

Fraumeri, J. F., ed. *Persons at High Risk of Cancer*. Academic Press, 1975.

Fritsch, A., ed. Center for Science in the Public Interest. *The Household Pollutants Guide*. Anchor Books, 1978.

Fry, J., and G. Fryers. *The Health Care Manual*. MTP Press, 1983.

Gear, Alan. *The New Organic Food Guide*. Dent, 1987.

Gibbs, A. *Understanding Mental Health*. Consumers' Association/Hodder & Stoughton, 1986.

Gibson, S. L. M., L. Templeton and R. G. Gibson. *Cook Yourself a Favour*. Thorsons, 1986.

Gordon, B. *I'm Dancing as Fast as I Can*. Bantam Books, 1980.

Grant, E. *The Bitter Pill: How Safe is the "Perfect Contraceptive"?* Elm Tree Books, 1985.

Hanssen, M. *E for Additives*. Thorsons, 1984.

Johnson, C., and A. Melville. *Hay Fever: No Need to Suffer*. Corgi, 1985.

Kidman, B. *A Gentle Way with Cancer*. Century, 1983.

Kilmartin, A. *Cystitis*. Warner Books, 1984.

Kitzinger, S. *Birth at Home*. Oxford University Press, 1979.

————. *The Experience of Childbirth*. Penguin, 1968.

La Croix, A. Z., et al. "Coffee consumption and coronary heart disease." *New England Journal of Medicine* 315 (1986): 977–978.

MacGregor, G. A. "Dietary sodium and potassium and blood pressure." *The Lancet*, April 2, 1983.

Mackarness, R. *Chemical Victims*. Stein & Day, 1980.

————. *Not All in the Mind*. Pan, 1976.

Margarian, G. J. "Hyperventilation syndromes: infrequently recognized common expressions of anxiety and stress." *Medicine* 61 (1982): 219–236.

Martindale, William, ed. *The Extra Pharmacopoeia*, 28th ed. Rittenhouse, 1983.

McKeown, T. *The Role of Medicine*. Princeton University Press, 1980.

Meadows, D. H., D. L. Meadows, J. Randers and W. W. Behrens. *The Limits to Growth*. New American Library, 1974.

Meares, A. *Relief Without Drugs*. Fontana, 1967.

Meirik, O., et al. "Joint national case-control study of breast cancer in Sweden and Norway." *The Lancet*, September 20, 1986.

Melville, A., and C. Johnson. *Cured to Death*. Stein & Day, 1983.

————. *The Long-Life Heart*. Century, 1985.

————. *Fat Free Forever*. Crown, 1987.

Mervyn, L. *Minerals and Your Health*. Keats, 1984.

Millstone, Erik. *Food Additives: Taking the Lid Off What We Really Eat.* Penguin, 1986.

Montgomery, E. *Regaining Bladder Control.* John Wright & Sons, 1974.

Nicolson, R. S. "Association of Public Analysts' Surveys of Pesticide Residues in Food, 1983." *Journal of the Association of Public Analysts* 22 (1984): 51–57.

Nixon, P. G. F. "Stress and the cardiovascular system." *The Practitioner* 226 (1982): 1589–1598.

_____. *Stress, life-style, and cardiovascular disease: a cardiological odyssey.* Paper presented to British Holistic Medical Association, 1983.

Orbach, S. *Fat Is a Feminist Issue.* Berkley, 1984.

Parish, P. *Medicines: A Guide for Everybody,* 5th ed. Penguin, 1986.

Passwater, R. A., and E. M. Cranton. *Trace Elements, Hair Analysis and Nutrition.* Keats, 1983.

Paul, A. A., and D. A. T. Southgate. *McCance & Widdowson's The Composition of Foods,* 4th ed. Elsevier, 1978.

Pfeiffer, C. C. *Zinc and Other Micro-Nutrients.* Keats, 1978.

Rands, D. A., and R. C. Godfrey. "Side effects of desensitization for allergy—a general practice survey." *Journal of the Royal College of General Practitioners* 33 (1983).

Rose, C. *Pesticides: The First Incidents Report.* Friends of the Earth, 1985.

Royal Canadian Air Force. *Physical Fitness.* Penguin, 1986.

Royal College of General Practitioners. *Trends in Morbidity in General Practice.* Royal College of General Practitioners, Occasional Paper No. 3, 1976.

Schell, O. *Modern Meat: Antibiotics, Hormones, and the Pharmaceutical Farm.* Random House, 1984.

Shephard, R. J. *Ischaemic Heart Disease and Exercise.* Croom Helm, 1981.

Simonton, O. C., S. Matthew-Simonton and J. L. Creighton. *Getting Well Again.* Cancer Control Society, 1978.

Stanley, N. F., and R. A. Joske. *Changing Disease Patterns and Human Behavior.* Academic Press, 1985.

Stanway, A. *Overcoming Depression.* Hamlyn, 1981.

_____. *Prevention is Better. . . .* David & Charles, 1987.

Steel, M. *Understanding Allergies.* Consumers' Association, 1986.

Sterling, A., et al. "Building Illness in the White-collar Workplace." *International Journal of Health Services* 13 (1983): 227–287.

Stoddard, A. *The Back: Relief from Pain.* Martin Dunitz, 1984.

Taylor, B., et al. "Breast feeding, eczema, asthma, and hayfever." *Journal of Epidemiology and Community Health* 37 (1983): 95–99.

Tollison, C. D. *Managing Chronic Pain: A Patient's Guide.* Sterling, 1982.

Trowell, H., and D. Burkitt, eds. *Western Diseases: Their Emergence and Prevention.* Harvard University Press, 1981.

Vessey, M. P., and M. Gray. *Cancer Risks and Prevention.* Oxford University Press, 1985.

Waldbott, G. C. *Health Effects of Environmental Pollutants.* 2nd ed. C. V. Mosby, 1978.

Watts, J. *An Investigation into the Use and Effects of Pesticides in the UK.* Friends of the Earth, 1985.

Wickett, W. H. *Herpes: Cause and Control.* Pinnacle, 1982.

Wilcox, R. G., et al. "Is exercise good for high blood pressure?" *British Medical Journal* 285 (1982): 767–769.

Wilkinson, M. *Migraine and Headaches.* Arco, 1982.

Wolff, M. S. "Occupationally derived chemicals in breast milk." *American Journal of Industrial Medicine* 4 (1983): 259–281.

Wynn, M., and A. Wynn. *Prevention of Handicap and the Health of Women.* Routledge & Kegan Paul, 1979.

Young, S., S. Shulman, and M. Shulman. *The Asthma Handbook.* Bantam Books, 1985.

Ziff, S. *Silver Dental Fillings: The Toxic Time Bomb.* Aurora, 1984.

INDEX OF
DRUG NAMES

Accurbron, 92
Acebutolol, 138
Acetaco, 70
Acetaminophen, 70, 72, 192, 203, 231
acetohexamide, 160–61
Achromycin, 75
Actidil, 85
Actifed, 72, 85
acyclovir, 246–47
Adapin, 47
Adipex-P, 166
Advil, 202
Advil Ibuprofen, 71
Aerolate, 92
Aeroseb-Dex, 87
Afrin, 85
Afrin Nasal Spray, 73, 86
Afrinol, 85
Agoral, 127, 128
A-hydroCort, 87
Akineton, 63
Alba-Temp, 70, 300
Aldactazide, 146
Aldactone, 146
Aldoclor, 146, 147
Aldomet, 147
Aldoril, 146, 147
Algisin, 70
Alka-Mints, 118
Alka-Seltzer, 70, 118
Alka Seltzer Plus Cold Medicine, 72
Allerest, 72, 85
allopurinol, 216
Alpha-Phed, 70
alprazolam, 53
Aludrox, 118
A-methaPred, 87
amiloride hydrochloride, 146
Aminophylline, 92
amitriptyline, 47

Amoxil, 74
Amoxycillin, 74
amphetamine, 31, 37, 62
Amphojel, 118
ampicillin, 74, 181
Anacin, 70
Anacin-3, 70
Analpram-HC, 132
Anaprox, 202
Antrocol, 120
Anturane, 216
Anusol, 131–32
Anusol-HC, 132
Apresazide, 146
Apresoline-Esidrix, 146
Aquaphyllin, 92
Aquatensen, 146
Aralen, 218
Aristocort, 87
Arthritis Pain Formula, 201
Asbron, 92
Ascriptin, 70
aspirin, 26, 35, 70–71, 77, 97, 109, 112, 192, 197, 201–2, 216, 231–32, 256, 260
Atarax, 53
atenolol, 138
Ativan, 53
Atrohist LA, 120
Atromid-S, 143
atropine, 120
Augmentin, 74
aurothioglucose, 218
Ayerst Epitrate, 92
Azo Gantanol, 75

bacampicillin, 74
B-A-C Tablets, 70
Bactrim, 75
Bancap HC, 70
Bayer Aspirin, 70

BC Powder, 70
beclomethasone dipropionate, 87
Beclovent Inhaler, 87
Beconase Inhaler, 87
Beconase Nasal Spray, 87
Belladenal, 120
belladonna, 120, 197
Bellergal-S, 197
Benadryl, 72, 85
Benadryl Anti-Itch Cream, 109
Bendectin, 256
bendroflumethiazide, 146
Benemid, 216
Bentyl, 120
Benzedrex Inhaler, 73, 86
benztropine, 63
benzylpenicillin, 74
betamethasone, 87, 107
Beta-Phed, 70
Betatrex, 107
Bicillin, 74
biperiden, 63
Blocadren, 138
Bromfed, 72
Broncholate, 92
Bronkodyl, 92
Bucet, 70
Bufferin, 70, 201
bumetanide, 146
Bumex, 146
Butazolidin, 202
Butisol Sodium, 59

Cafergot, 197
caffeine, 30, 31, 33, 58
Calan, 138–39
Cama Arthritis Pain Reliever, 201
Camalox, 118
Capoten, 147

329

Capozide, 146, 147
captopril, 147–48
CardeCort, 107
Carisoprodol, 70
Carmol-HC, 132
Carter's Little Pills, 127
Catapres, 147, 197
Celestone, 87
Centrax, 53
Cerose-DM, 72
Chenix, 177
Chexit, 70
chlopropamide, 160–61
Chloral hydrate, 58
Chloraseptic, 71
chlordiazepoxide, 53
chlormezanone, 53
Chloroquine, 218
chlorothiazide, 146
chlorpromazine, 62
chlorprothixene, 62
chlorthalidone, 146
Chlor-Trimeton, 72, 85
cholestyramine, 143–44
cimetidine, 120
Cinomide, 87
Citrucel, 128
Clinoril, 202
clobetasol, 107
clofibrate, 143
clonazepam, 53
clonidine (hydrochloride),
147, 197
clorazepate, 53
clotrimazole, 243
cloxacillin, 74
cocaine, 35, 37, 38, 62
Codalan, 70
codeine, 73, 112
Cogentin, 63
Co-Gesic, 70
Colace, 128
Colestid, 143
colestipol, 143–44
Col-Probenecid, 216
Combipres, 146, 147
Compazine, 62, 123
Comtrex, 70, 72, 85
Comtrex Multi-symptom
Cold Reliever, 72
Congespirin for Children,
70, 72
Constant-T, 92
Contac, 72
Corgard, 138
Coricidin, 70, 72, 85
Coricidin D, 72
Coricidin Decongestant
Nasal Mist, 73, 86
Correctol, 128
Correctol Natural Grain, 128

Correctol tablets, 127
Cortaid, 107
Cort-Dome, 105, 132
Cortifoam, 132
cortisone acetate, 87
Cortisporin, 105
Cortone, 87
Cortril, 105
Corzide, 146
Co-Tylenol Cold Medication,
72
cromolyn sodium, 86, 91
Cuprimine, 218
Cyklokapron, 87

Daladone, 87
Dalmane, 58
Darvocet-N, 202
Darvon, 202, 203
Datril, 70
Decadron, 87
Decaspray, 87
Decholin, 177
Delacort, 85, 107
Deltasone, 87
Demazin, 72, 85
Demi-Regroton, 146, 147
Depen, 218
Depo-Medrol, 87
Deponit NTG Film, 139
Depo-Predate, 87
Deprol, 53
desipramine, 47
desonide, 107
DesOwen, 107
Desyrel, 47
dexamethasone, 87
Dexasone, 87
Dextromethorphan, 73–74
Diabenese, 160–61
Dialose, 128
Dialose Plus, 127
diazepam, 53
diazoxide, 147
Dibenyline, 147
dichloralphenazone, 58
dicyclomine, 120
diethylpropion, 166
diflunisal, 202
digitalis, 26
Dilatrate, 139
diltiazem, 139
Dimetane, 72, 85
Dimetapp, 70, 72, 85
diphenoxylate, 125
Diprolene, 107
Diprosone, 107
Disipal, 85
Disophrol, 85
Diucardin, 146

Diulo, 146
Diupres, 146, 147
Diuril, 146
Dolacet, 70
Dolene, 202
Dolobid, 202
Donnagel, 120, 231
Donnagel-PG, 118, 120
Donnatal, 120, 231
Dorcol Children's, 70
doxepin, 47
Dristal, 86
Dristan, 72, 73, 85
Drixoral, 70, 72, 85
droperidol, 62
Dulcolax, 127
Duocet, 70
Duotrate, 139
Duraphyl, 92
Duration 12-Hour Nasal
Spray, 73, 86
Dyazide, 146
Dyrenium, 146

Easprin, 70
Ecotrin, 70
Ecotrin Enteric Coated
Aspirin, 201
Edecrin, 146
Effer-syllium, 128
Elavil, 47
Elixophyllin, 92
Empirin, 70
Emulsoil, 127
enalapril, 148
Endep, 47
Eno, 118
epinephrine, 72, 91–92
EpiPen, 92
Equagesic, 53
Equanil, 53
Ergomar, 197
ergotamine tartrate,
197
erythromycin, 105
Esgic, 70
Esidrix, 146
Esimil, 146, 147
Eskalith, 48
ethacrynic acid, 146
Etrafon, 47, 62
Evac-U-Gen, 127
Excedrin, 70
Ex-Lax, 127
Extra Gentle Ex-Lax, 128

famotidine, 120
Fedahist, 72, 85
Feen-a-Mint, 127, 128
Feldene, 202
fenfluramine, 166

Fiberall, 128
Fibercon, 128
Fioricet, 70
Fiorinal, 70
fluphenazine, 62
flurazepam, 58
Fototar Cream, 112
4-Way Nasal Spray, 73, 86
Fungizone, 114
Furadantin, 181
furosemide, 146

Ganatol, 75
Gaviscon, 118
Gelpirin, 70
Gelusil, 118
Gentle Nature Natural
    Vegetable Laxative, 127
Geriplex-FS, 128
glipizide, 160–61
Glucotrol, 160–61
gold sodium thiomalate,
    218
G-1 Capsules, 70
guanethidine, 147
Gyne-Lotrimin, 243

Halcion, 58
Haldol, 62
Haley's M-O, 118, 127,
    128
haloperidol, 62
Haltran, 71
Hexadrol, 87
H-H-R, 146
H2-Blockers, 120–21
Humulin, 160
Hydeltrasol, 87
hydralazine, 147
Hydra-zide, 146
Hydrisalic Gel, 112
hydrochlorothiazide, 146
Hydrocil, 128
hydrocortisone, 87
Hydrocortisone cream, 105,
    107
Hydrocortone, 87
HydroDIURIL, 146
hydroflumethiazide, 146
Hydromox, 147
Hydropres, 146, 147
hydroxyzine, 53
Hygroton, 146

ibuprofen, 71, 97, 192, 202,
    231–32
Iletin, 160
Iletin Lente, 160
Iletin Semilente, 160
Iletin Ultralente, 160
imipramine, 41

Inapsine, 62
indapamide, 146
Inderal, 54, 138
Inderide, 138, 146
Indocin, 202, 216
indomethacin, 202, 216
Innovar, 62
insulin, 159–63
Insulin Injection USP, 160
Intal, 86, 91
Ionamin, 166
Ismelin, 147
isocarboxazid, 48
Isocom, 58, 197
Isometheptene mucate,
    197
Isoptin, 138–39
Isordil, 139
isosorbide dinitrate, 139
Isotrate Timecelles, 139

kaolin, 118, 125
Kasof, 128
Kemadrin, 63
Kenalog, 87
ketoprofen, 202

labetalol, 138
Lasix, 146
Lente Insulin, 160
Librax, 53
Libritol, 47
Librium, 53
Liquid Pred Syrup, 87
Liquiprin, 70
Lithane, 48
lithium carbonate, 48–49
lithium citrate, 48–49
Lithobid, 48
Loniten, 147
Lopressor, 138
Lopressor HCT, 138, 146
Lopurin, 216
lorazepam, 53
Lorcet, 70, 202
Lorelco, 143
Lortab, 70
Lortab ASA, 70
lotrimin cream, 114, 248
Lotrisone, 107
Lozol, 146
Ludiomil, 47
Lurline, 70

Maalox, 118
Macrodantin, 181
Maltsupex, 128
maprotiline, 47
Marax, 53, 91, 92
marijuana, 34, 35–36, 123,
    154

Marplan, 48
Maximum Strength Midol,
    197
Maxivate, 107
Maxzide, 146
Mazanor, 166
Mazindol, 166
Medicone, 131–32
Medigesic Plus, 70
Medihaler-Epi, 92
Medipren, 71, 202
Medrol, 87
mefenamic acid, 202
MegaMor, 70
Mellaril, 62
meprobamate, 53
Meprospan, 53
Metamucil, 128
Metatensin, 147
methyclothiazide, 146
methylcellulose, 125, 129,
    166
methyldopa, 147
methylprednisolone, 87
methysergide, 197
metolazole, 146
metoprolol, 138
miconazole, 244
Midamor, 146
Midol 200, 71, 202
Midrin, 58, 70, 197
Migralam, 70, 197
Milkinol, 128
Milk of Magnesia, 118, 127,
    247
Miltown, 53
Minipress, 147
Minizide, 146, 147
minoxidil, 147
Modane, 127
Moduretic, 146
Momentum Muscular
    Backache Formula, 201
Monistat, 243
Monistat-Derm, 114
Mordane Versabran, 128
Motrin, 71, 202
Mudrane GG Elixir, 91, 92
Mudrane Tablets, 92
Mycelex, 243, 248
Mycelex Cream, 114
Mycostatin, 243
Mylanta, 118
Myochrysine, 218
Mysteclin, 75

nadolol, 138
Naldecon CX Adult Liquid,
    74
Naprosyn, 202
naproxen, 202, 232

Naquival, 147
Nardil, 48
Nasalcrom, 86
Nature's Remedy, 127
Naturetin, 146
Nembutal, 59
Neoloid, 127
Neosporin, 105
Neo-Synephrine, 73, 86–87
Nephrox, 118
Neucalm, 53
Nilstat, 243
Nipride, 147
Nitro-Bid, 139
Nitrocine, 139
Nitrodisc, 139
Nitro-Dur, 139
nitrofurantoin, 181
Nitrogard Buccal Tablets,
    139
nitroglycerin, 139
Nitroglyn, 139
Nitrol IV, 139
Nitrolingual Spray, 139
Nitrong, 139
Nitropress, 147
Nitrospan, 139
Nitrostat, 139
Nodular, 59
Norgesic, 70
Normodyne, 138
Normozide, 138, 146
Norpramin, 47
nortriptyline, 47
Norwich Aspirin, 70
Nostril, 85
Nostrilla, 85
Nostril Nasal Decongestant,
    73, 87
Novahistine, 72, 85
Novolin, 160
NPH Iletin, 160
NPH Purified Pork Insulin,
    160
NT2, 73, 86
Nuprin, 202
Nuprin Ibuprofen, 71
nystatin, 244

Oby-Trim, 166
Omnipen, 74
opium, 31, 35, 73
Opticrom, 86
Orap, 62
Oretic, 146
Oreticil, 146
Original Formula Midol, 70,
    197
Orinase, 161
orphenadrine, 63
Orudis, 202

Otrivan, 73, 87
oxazepam, 53
oxytetracycline, 75

Pamelor, 47
Panadol, 70
Parepectolin, 118
Parnate, 48
penicillamine, 218
penicillin G, 74
penicillins, 20, 74–75, 78,
    79
penicillin V, 74
pentaerythritol tetranitrate,
    139
Pentids, 74
Pen-Vee K, 74
Pepcid, 120
Percocet, 70
Percodan, 70
Percogesic, 70
Perdiem Granules, 127, 128
Peritrate, 139
Permitil, 62
perphenazine, 62
Persistin, 70
Pertofrane, 47
P.E.T.N., 139
phenelzine, 48
Phenergan, 58–59
phenoxybenzamine
    hydrochloride, 147
phentermin, 166
phenylbutazone, 202
phenylephrine hydrochloride,
    72
Phillips' LaxCaps, 127, 128
Phrenilin, 70
pimozide, 62
pindolol, 138
piroxicam, 202
PMB 200, 53
PMB 400, 53
polythiazide, 146
Pondimin, 166
prazepam, 53
prazosin, 147
Predate 50, 87
Prediapred, 87
Prednicen-M, 87
prednisolone, 87
prednisone, 87
Prelone, 87
Pre-Pen, 74
Primatene, 92
Primatene Tablets (M and P
    Formulae), 91, 92
Principen, 74
Privine, 73, 87
Pro-Banthine, 120, 185
probucol, 143

prochlorperazine, 62
Proctofoam-HC, 132
Proctofoam/non-steroid,
    131–32
procyclidine, 63
progesterone, 227, 229
Proglycem, 147
Prolixin, 62
Proloprim, 75
promazine, 62
promethazine, 58–59
propantheline, 120, 185
propoxyphene, 202–3
propranolol, 54, 138
Protamine, 160
protriptyline, 47
pseudoephedrine
    hydrochloride, 72
Purge Concentrate, 127
Pyridium Plus, 59
Pyrroxate, 70, 72, 85

Quadrinal, 92
Quelidrine Syrup, 92
Questran, 143

ranitidine, 120
Raudixin, 147
Rauwiloid, 147
Rauzide, 146, 147
Regroton, 147
Regutol, 128
Renese, 146, 147
Repan, 70
reserpine, 147
Respbid, 92
Restoril, 58
Robaxisal, 70
Robitussin, 72
Robitussin Night Relief,
    72
Rolaids, 118
Roxicet, 70
Roxiprin, 70
Rufen, 71
Ryna-C, 74
Ryna-CX, 74
Ryna Liquid, 72, 85
Rynatuss, 92

salicylates, 97, 109
saline laxatives, 127
Saluron, 146
Salutensin, 146, 147
Sanorex, 166
Sansert, 197
scopolamine, 120, 231
Sedapap, 70
Seldane, 86
Semilente Insulin, 160

Septra, 75
Ser-Ap-Es, 146, 147
Serax, 53
Serpasil, 147
Serpasil-Esidrex, 146
Serutan, 128
Simeco, 118
Sinarest, 70, 85
Sine-Aid, 70
Sine-off, 72
Sinequan, 47
Singlet, 70, 72
Sinubid, 70
Sinulin, 70
Sinutab, 70, 72
Slo-bid, 92
Slo-Phyllin, 92
sodium nitroprusside, 147
Solganal, 218
Soma Compound, 70
Sominex, 70
Somphyllin, 92
Span R/D, 166
Spasgesic, 70
Spectazole Cream, 114
Spectrobid, 74
spironolactone, 146
Stelazine, 62, 123
Sterapred, 87
Sudafed, 72, 85
sulfamethizole, 75
Sulfamethoprim, 75
Sulfamethoxazole/ Trimethoprim, 75
sulfinpyrazone, 216
Sulfonamides, 74, 75, 181
sulindac, 202
Sumycin, 75
Supac, 70
Surfac, 128
Surmontil, 47
Sustaire, 92
Swan Citroma, 127
Syllact, 128
Synalgos-DC, 70

Tagamet, 120
Talacen, 70
Taracton, 62
T-Diet, 166
Tedral, 91, 92
Tedral Elixir, 92
Tedral Tablets, 92
Teldrin, 85
Temaril, 58–59
temazepam, 58
Temovate, 107

Tempra, 70
Tencet, 70
Tenoretic, 138, 146
Tenormin, 138
Tenuate, 166
Tepanil, 166
Teramine, 166
Terfenadine, 86
Terramycin, 75
tetracyclines, 74, 75, 104–5, 117, 181
Thalidone, 146
Theobid, 92
theobromine, 30–31, 33
Theochron, 92
Theoclear, 92
Theo-Dur, 92
Theofedral, 92
Theofedral Tablets, 91
Theolair, 92
Theon, 92
Theo-Organidin, 92
theophylline, 33, 91–92
Theospan-SR, 92
Theostat, 92
Theo-24, 92
Theovent, 92
thioridazine, 62
Thiosulfil, 75
Thorazine, 62, 123
thymol, 71
Timolide, 138, 146
timolol, 138
Tofranil, 47
tolazamide, 160–61
Tolbutamide, 161
Tolinase, 161
Topicycline, 75, 105
T-Quil, 53
Trancopal, 53
Trandate, 138
Trandate HCT, 146
Transderm-Nitro, 139
Tranxene, 53
tranylcypromine, 48
trazodone, 47
Trendar, 71
Triad, 70
triamcinolone, 87
Triaminic, 72, 85
triamterene, 146
Trianimicol, 72
Triavil, 47, 62
triazolam, 58
Tridesilon, 107
Tridil, 139
trifluoperazine, 62
Trilafon, 62
trimeprazine, 58–59

trimethoprim, 75
Triminicin, 70
trimipramine, 47
Trimox, 74
Trimpex, 75
Trisilate, 118
Tronolane, 131–32
Tums, 118
Tylenol, 70
Tylox, 70

Ultralente insulin, 160
Unasyn, 74
Uniphyl, 92
Unisom, 70
Urobiotic, 75
Ursinus, 70

Valisone, 107
Valium, 53
Valrelease, 53
Vancenase Inhaler, 87
Vanceril Inhaler, 87
Vanoxide-HC Acne Lotion, 105
Vanquish, 70
Vaponefrin, 92
Vaseretic, 146, 148
Vasotec, 148
Veetids, 74
Velosulin, 160
Velosulin Human, 160
verapamil, 138–39
Vicks Daycare, 72
Vicks Formula 44, 72
Vicks Nyquil, 72
Vicks Sinex, 73, 85, 87
Vicks Throat Lozenges, 71
Vistaril, 53
Vivactil, 47

Whitfield's Ointment, 112
Wigraine, 197
WinGel, 118
Wyanoids, 132
Wygesic, 70, 202
Wymox, 74

Xanax, 53

Yellowlax, 127

Zantac, 120
Zaroxolyn, 146
Zinc & Iletain I, 160
Zorprin, 70
Zovirax, 246–47
Zydone, 70
Zyloprim, 216

GENERAL INDEX

abdominal breathing, 93–94, 95
Accent on Information, 224
acne and spots, 104–6
Action on Smoking and Health, 79
activity, *see* exercise and activity
acupuncture, 26, 194
addiction, drug, 33–37, 202
adolescence, depression in, 45
adrenaline, 32
aggression, 34, 37
agoraphobia, 52, 54, 56–57
AIDS, 236, 245
alcohol, 30, 31, 34, 46, 71, 86, 150, 200,
    249
  digestive problems and, 119, 121, 126
  joint problems and, 216
  kidneys and, 180
  pregnancy and, 255, 260
  premenstrual syndrome and, 230
  sleep and, 60
allergies, 111, 173
  to chemicals, 46, 84, 97
  to drugs, 74–75, 84, 97
  food, *see* food allergies
  reduced susceptibility to, 98–99
  respiratory, *see* asthma; hay fever; perennial
    rhinitis; respiratory allergies
  respiratory infections and, 66, 74–75, 80
alternative (complementary) medicine, 11,
    12, 14, 15, 24–29
aluminum, 118
Alzheimer's disease, 118
American College of Home Obstetrics, 259
amino acids, 307
analgesics, 197, 216, 229, 231
angina, 118, 135, 137–42, 147
angioedema, *see* urticaria and angioedema
ankles, arthritis relief for, 223
antacids, 118, 120
antibiotics, 74–75, 78, 79, 104–5, 107, 117,
    126, 130, 177, 181
anticholinergic drugs, 120, 123, 129, 185,
    197

antidepressants, 47–49, 54, 197
  cold remedies and, 72–73
antihistamines, 19–20, 58–59, 72, 73, 85–
    86, 120–23
antipsychotics, 62–63, 120, 123
anxiety, 42, 51, 52, 57, 126, 249
  see also stress management
arteries, hardening of, 142–43
arthritis, 214, 217–24
Arthritis Foundation, 224
artificial sweeteners, 31, 164, 167
asthma, 71, 82, 84, 90–98, 125, 192
atherosclerosis and atheroma, 142–43

back care products, 212–13
back pain, 209–13
bacteria, 68, 74, 75, 117, 126
  cystitis and, 181
  skin infections and, 113
balanced life-style, 136, 157, 314
barbiturates, 31, 59
bed-wetting, 184–86
benzodiazepines, 53, 54, 58
Beta blockers, 20, 54, 97, 138, 145, 154,
    197
birth, *see* pregnancy and birth
Birth at Home (Kitzinger), 259
birth control, *see* contraception, drugs for
birth defects, 252, 255–56
Bitter Pill, The (Grant), 235
bladder, 172–73, 183, 185, 186–88
blood pressure, 267
  drugs for, 46, 145–48
  increase in, 32, 72, 148; *see also*
    hypertension
blood-vessel disease, *see* cardiovascular disease
bowel habits, 129
brain, 43–45, 86
breast cancer, 236
breast-feeding, 110, 262
breathing, 199
  asthma and, 93–94, 95
  cardiovascular disease and, 140–41

pain relief and, 195
  stress and, 52, 53, 57, 61, 274, 278–79
breathlessness, asthma and, 90–91
British National Formulary, 244, 256
bronchitis, 66, 67, 69, 74, 75, 79–80
bronchodilators, 91–92
bulking agents, 126, 128
bursitis, 214–15
B vitamins, 165, 175, 252, 254, 303–4
  see also specific vitamins
Byrivers, Patricia, 219

calcium, 118, 180
calcium antagonists, 138–39
calcium oxalates, 179–80
cancer, 29, 34, 236, 255
  cervical, 33, 245, 248
  treatment of, 36, 46, 123, 124
candidiasis (vaginal thrush; yeast infection),
  130, 243–45, 307–8
Cannon, G., 308
carbohydrates, 242
  complex, 51, 119, 164
  sleep and, 60–61
cardiovascular disease, 35, 52, 72–73, 120,
  133–55, 270–71
  see also specific cardiovascular diseases
cardiovascular system, 134–37
Centers for Disease Control, 33
cervical cancer, 33, 245, 248
chemicals, 182, 255
  allergies to, 46, 84, 97
  infertility and, 238–39
chilblains, 153–55
Childbirth Without Pain Association, 258
children, 45, 88
  asthma in, 82, 96, 97–98
  bed-wetting of, 184–86
  diabetes of, 158, 159
  digestive problems of, 124, 125, 126
  respiratory infections of, 66, 67, 71, 75, 77
  skin disorders of, 110–11
chiropractors, 25–26
chocolate, 33, 119, 199
cholecystitis, 177
cholesterol, 141, 143–44
chromium, 162, 164, 303, 306
chronic pain, 200–208
cigarette smoking, *see* smoking
cirrhosis, 34
claustrophobia, 52
clothing, 114, 154, 182, 188, 244–45
cocoa, 31, 33
coffee, 30, 33, 58, 60, 185, 199, 200, 253
  asthma and, 92
  digestive problems and, 119, 121, 126
  liver problems and, 175, 176
  premenstrual syndrome and, 230

cola drinks, 31, 33, 119, 185, 230
colds, 66, 69, 72–73, 75–77, 84, 97, 109
cold sores (herpes), 112–13, 246–48
colon, spastic (irritable bowel syndrome),
  129–30
Comfort, Alex, 239
complementary medicine, *see* alternative
  medicine
condoms, 236, 245
constipation, 125–29, 131, 188, 232
contraception, drugs for, 235–37
  see also specific forms of contraception
copper, 220
co-trimoxazole, 74, 75, 79, 105
cough mixtures, 73–74, 97, 109
coughs, 69, 79–80
counseling, 281
crack, 31, 37, 38
cramps, leg, 152–53
Crohn's disease, 130–31
culture, drugs and, 30, 31, 35, 37–38
Cured to Death (Melville and Johnson), 12
cysteine, 307
cystitis, 173, 180–84

dancing, 287–88
decongestant sprays, 72, 73, 86–87
dehydration, 126, 200
Depo-Provera, 235
depression, 36, 37, 41–42, 45–51, 53, 147
  duration of, 41, 45–46
  insomnia and, 42, 51, 57
  serotonin and, 44, 45, 51
dermatitis, *see* rashes and dermatitis
DES (diethylstilbestrol), 256
desensitization, 56–57, 88–89
detergents, 100, 108, 182
diabetes, 20, 46, 71, 157–64, 249
  cardiovascular disease and, 142
  cold remedies and, 72–73
  digestive problems and, 123, 124, 163
Diane, 105
diaphragms, 236
diarrhea, 124–26, 129, 131
diet:
  cardiovascular disease and, 141–44, 154
  cystitis and, 183
  depression and, 46, 51
  digestive problems and, 119, 121–22, 130,
    131
  elimination, 308–9
  fats in, 298–300
  gallbladder problems and, 178
  headaches and, 198, 199, 200
  infertility and, 238–39
  joint problems and, 216–17, 219–20
  kidneys and, 179
  liver problems and, 175–76

diet (*continued*)
  metabolism problems and, 162–65, 167, 168
  in pregnancy, 98, 251–54, 257
  premenstrual syndrome and, 229–30
  respiratory allergies and, 98–99
  respiratory infections and, 76–77, 80
  skin disorders and, 105, 109–12, 114
  sleep and, 60–61
  stress and, 55–56
dieting, 199, 235, 251, 296
Dieting Makes You Fat (Cannon and Enzig), 308
digestive problems, 115–32
  see also specific digestive problems
digestive system, 116–17
diuretics, 33, 145–46, 185, 186, 216, 229
diverticulitis, 130–31
doctors:
  education of, 21
  malpractice suits feared by, 20–21
  prescriptions of, 22–23
Dohan, Curtis, 64
Dong, Dr., 220
douching, 242–43
drainage methods, 94
Dr. Dong's Arthritis Cookbook, 220
drug abuse, legal vs. illegal, 31
drug addiction, 31, 33–37, 202
drug companies, 21–22, 32
drugs:
  allergies to, 74–75, 84, 97
  dangers of, 10–14, 19–23
  defined, 30
  digestive problems and, 122
  everyday, 30–38
  exporting of, 22, 33
  good and appropriate use of, 14, 23
  herbal remedies compared with, 26–27
  illicit, 35–37
  increased use of, 9, 10
  as magic bullet, 23
  over-the-counter (OTCs), 33, 34–35
  regulation of, 22
  side effects of, 12, 19–21
  street illegal, 31, 35–37
  testing of, 13, 20
Drugs Anonymous, 54
duodenum, 116, 120

earache, 74, 78
East West Journal, 302
Eating Dangerously (Mackarness), 46, 309
eczema, 110–11, 125
Ehrlich, Paul, 23
elderly, 54, 63
  respiratory infections of, 66, 71
  sleeping patterns of, 59–60

electroconvulsive therapy (ECT), 63
emotions:
  destructive, 151
  distress and, 41–65
  suppression of, 196
Enzig, H., 308
Eraldin, 22
esophagus, 116, 117
estrogen, 227, 233–34
exercise and activity, 51, 55, 61, 106, 283–95
  asthma and, 94–95
  for bladder and pelvic floor, 187
  cardiovascular disease and, 140, 143, 150–54
  digestive problems and, 128, 130
  headaches and, 199
  joint problem relief and, 220–23
  liver problems and, 176–77
  menstrual pain and, 232
  metabolic problems and, 163–64, 168–69
  pain relief and, 194, 199, 203–4, 211–12
  pregnancy and, 254
  premenstrual syndrome and, 230
  Royal Canadian Air Force (RCAF) workout, 129, 290, 291, 294
exercises, mental, pain-control and, 207–8
exhaustion, 269–72
Experience of Childbirth, The (Kitzinger), 258

faith healers, 27–28
Fat Free Forever (Melville and Johnson), 175, 200
Fat Is a Feminist Issue (Orbach), 170
fats, dietary, 298–300
fatty acids, essential, 99, 130, 299–300, 306–7
fecal softeners, 128
feet, cold, 153–55
fiber, dietary, 180
  digestive problems and, 122, 126, 128, 130, 131
  foods high in, 302–3
fish oils, 144
Five-Day Plan to Stop Smoking, 79–80
flu, 46, 67, 69, 75–76
folic acid, 175, 253, 304
follicle-stimulating hormone, 227
food:
  asthma and, 97
  high-fiber, 302–3
  organic, 300–302, 321–24
  processed, 32, 99, 200
  see also diet
food additives, 32, 97, 310–12
food allergies, 46, 62, 97, 98–99, 117
  arthritis and, 219–20
  cystitis and, 183

digestive problems and, 125, 130
elimination diets and, 308–9
headaches and, 200
schizophrenia and, 64
Food and Drug Administration (FDA), 20, 22
Fritsch, A., 176
function curve, heart attack and, 270–71
fungal infections, of the skin, 113, 114

gallbladder, 116, 117–18, 172–73, 177–78
gamma-linoleic acid (GLA), 229–30, 232, 233, 234
gastroenteritis, 35
Goodbye to Arthritis (Byrivers), 219
Gordon, Barbara, 53
gout, 216–17
Grant, Ellen, 235

hands:
  arthritis relief for, 222
  cold, 153–55
hay fever, 82, 85–90, 98, 125
headaches, 192, 195–200
  migraine, 196–99
  tension, 195–96
health, 313–16
  defined, 10
  drugs and, 10–14, 19–23
  holistic approach to, 13–14, 28–29
  illness vs., 11–14, 24, 28–29
heart:
  drugs for, 46
  see also cardiovascular disease
heartburn, *see* indigestion and heartburn
Help for Incontinent People, 188
hemorrhoids, 131–32
hepatitis, 173
herbal remedies, 26–27
hernia, hiatal, 117
heroin, 31, 37, 38
herpes (cold sores), 112–13, 246–48
hips, arthritis relief for, 222–23
histamines, 84, 86
holistic approach, 13–14, 28–29
homeopathy, 25
hormones, 135, 308
  corticosteriod, 87–88
  in menstrual cycle, 227, 229
  migraines and, 198, 199
  replacement therapy and, 157
  skin disorders and, 105, 106, 112
Household Pollutant Guide, The (Fritsch), 176
hygiene, 100, 108, 111
  cystitis and, 182–83
  vaginitis and vulvovaginitis and, 241–42
hyperlipidemia (high blood cholesterol), 143–144
hypertension (high blood pressure), 142–52

hypoglycemia, 119, 160, 163, 164–65
hysterectomies, 46

iatrogenic disease, 12, 20–21
illness:
  drug-induced, 12, 20–21
  health vs., 11–14, 24, 28–29
  during pregnancy, 254
  symptom treating vs. cure of, 22, 23
I'm Dancing as Fast as I Can (Gordon), 53
immune systems, 68–69, 80–81, 172–73
  allergies and, 83–84, 98
immunotherapy, 88–89
impotence, 248–49
indigestion and heartburn, 117–19
infections:
  antihistamines and, 86
  improved immunity to, 80–81
  steroids and, 92–93
  see also specific infections
infertility, 237–40
inflammatory bowel disease, 130–31
Information Center for Individuals with Disabilities, 224
insomnia, 33, 42, 51, 57–61
interferons, 68, 69, 76
International Association for Childbirth at Home, 259
Interstitial Cystitis Association, 184
intestines, 116–17, 122
ionizers, 100–101
iron, 117, 175, 220, 234, 253, 305
irritable bowel syndrome (spastic colon), 129–130
IUDs, 231, 233, 236–37, 238, 245–46

jaundice, 174
joint problems, 214–24
  bursitis, 214–15
  gout, 216–17
  see also arthritis
Joy of Sex, The (Comfort), 239

kidney disease, 178–79
kidneys, 34, 35, 70, 172–73, 179
kidney stones, 179–80
Kitzinger, Sheila, 258, 259
knees, arthritis relief for, 223

labor, 259–62
laxatives, 126–29
legs:
  restless or cramped, 152–53
  ulcers of, 114, 152–53
lifting, back pain and, 210–11
liver, 33, 34, 172–77, 192
  drug side effects and, 35, 70
liver disease, 117–18, 173–74

LSD (d-lysergic acid diethylamide), 36–37, 62
lubricant laxatives, 127–28
luteinizing hormone, 227
lymph glands, 69

Mackarness, Richard, 46, 309
McKeown, Thomas, 313–14
magnesium, 118, 127, 162, 180, 306
    cardiovascular disease and, 141–42, 154
    premenstrual syndrome and, 230
manganese, 162, 306
Medicines (Parish), 73
meditation, 276
Melzack, Ron, 194
men:
    herpes in, 246–47
    impotence in, 248–49
    infertility and, 237–40
    penis infections of, 248
    stress in, 271–72
    vasectomy in, 237
    vitamin C and, 77
menstrual pain, 36, 193, 227, 231–33
menstruation, menstrual cycle, 226–35
    see also premenstrual syndrome
metabolism, 31, 34, 112, 156–70, 199, 309–310
    see also diabetes; hypoglycemia; obesity
methionine, 307
migraine headaches, 196–99
milk, 126, 253
minerals, 27, 253
    see also specific minerals
mite, house-dust, 99–100
mold spores, 96
monoamine oxidase inhibitors (MAOIs), 48, 73
mononucleosis, 46
monosodium glutamate (MSG), 200, 220
morning sickness, drugs for, 256
motion sickness, 124
muscle relaxation, 277–78
mutagens, 254

nausea and vomiting, 123–26, 163
neck, arthritis relief for, 222
nerve stimulation, 194, 208
nervous system, cardiovascular disease and, 135, 138
neurosis, 42, 52
neurotransmitters, 44–45, 47, 48, 51
niacin (nicotinic acid), 162, 164, 303–4
nicotine, 31, 33–34, 154, 252
Nixon, Peter, 270–71
nonsteroidal anti-inflammatories (NSAIs), 201–2, 217–18

norepinephrine, 45
nose drops, 72, 73, 86–87

obesity, 117, 136, 150, 165–70
obsessions, 42, 52, 294
oral contraceptives, 46, 105, 198, 227, 232, 235–36, 238, 244, 262
Orbach, Susie, 170
organic foods, 300–302, 321–24
orthomolecular medicine, 27
osteoarthritis, see arthritis
osteopaths, 25–26
ovulation, 227–28, 238, 239

pain, 189–213
    back, 209–13
    cardiovascular disease and, 135, 137–42
    chronic, 200–208
    of earache, 78
    insomnia and, 57–58
    menstrual, 36, 193, 227, 231–33
    minor, 192–94
pain-relieving drugs, 70–71, 72
panic attacks, 52, 54–55, 278–79
Parish, Peter, 73
Parkinson's disease, 46, 63
pelvic inflammatory disease (PID), 237, 246
penis, infections of, 248
peptic ulcers, 71, 119–23
perennial rhinitis, 82, 85–90
pesticides, 32, 100, 173
phobias, 42, 52, 54, 56–57
Physicians' Desk Reference (PDR), 91, 112, 147, 249
pituitary gland, 233
plateauing, exercise and, 294
pneumonia, 69, 74
pollution, 80–81, 97–98
    reduction of, 100–101
positive thinking, pain relief and, 205–7
posture, 195–96, 209–10
potassium, 127, 146, 149, 306
pregnancy and birth, 98, 117, 132, 250–62
    drugs and, 71, 75, 192, 252, 254–58
    healthy, 252–54
    illness during, 254
    labor and, 259–62
    medicalization of, 257–58
    preparing for, 251–52, 258–59
premenstrual syndrome (PMS), 46, 199, 227–31, 233, 234, 308
prostaglandins, 201
protein, kidney problems and, 180
psoriasis, 111–12
psychotherapy, 63
Public Citizen Health Research Group, 202
pyridoxine (vitamin B$_6$), 51, 180, 229, 253, 257, 304

rashes and dermatitis, 106–8
Raynaud's disease, 153–55
relationships, depression and, 46, 51
relaxation, 55, 61, 124, 273–79
    asthma and, 95–96
    breathing and, 274, 278–79
    cardiovascular disease and, 140, 149, 150
    muscle, 277–78
    pain relief and, 193–95, 198, 203
reproductive system, 225–49
    see also contraception
respiratory allergies, 82–101
    see also asthma; hay fever; perennial rhinitis
respiratory infections, 66–81
    see also specific respiratory infections
respiratory system, 67–68
Reye's Syndrome, 71, 77, 192
rheumatism, 214
    see also arthritis
Role of Medicine, The (McKeown), 313–14
Royal Canadian Air Force (RCAF) workout,
    129, 290, 291, 294
running, 290–92

salt, 32, 149–50, 253, 312
sanitary napkins, 243, 247
schizophrenia, 37, 42, 62–64
sebum, 103, 104
sedatives, 43, 46, 47, 58–59, 186, 256
serotonin, 44–45, 51
sexual behavior, sex, 34, 37, 61, 204, 281
    cystitis and, 182, 183–84
    impotence and, 248–49
    infertility and, 239–40
    lubrication and, 242
    skin disorders and, 105
shoulders, arthritis relief in, 222
Simon Foundation, 188
sitting, back pain and, 210
skin disorders, 102–14
    see also specific skin disorders
sleep, 275
    back pain and, 210
    see also insomnia
SmokEnders, 80
smoking, 33–34, 100, 303
    back pain and, 209
    cardiovascular disease and, 133–34, 141,
        142, 143, 153
    digestive problems and, 119, 122
    leg ulcers and, 114
    liver problems and, 175, 176
    pregnancy and, 252
    quitting, 79–80
    respiratory infections and, 66–67, 78–81
    skin disorders and, 106
    stress and, 268
soap, 100, 108, 111, 182, 241–42

sodium, 32, 127, 149–50
sore throats, 66, 71, 77
spas, 95–96
spastic colon (irritable bowel syndrome), 129–
    130
spermicides, 236, 241
Stanway, Andrew, 45
sterilization, 237
steroids, 87–88, 92 -93, 107–8, 110, 112,
    122, 130, 131, 132, 157, 218
stimulant laxatives, 127
stomach, 71, 116, 119, 120, 122
stress, 32, 52–57, 72
    bed-wetting and, 85–86
    cardiovascular disease and, 135–36, 139,
        140, 144, 151
    digestive problems and, 122–23, 125, 130
    exhaustion and, 269–72
    herpes and, 247
    hypoglycemia and, 165
    impotence and, 249
    infection and, 81
    infertility and, 240
    menstrual cycle and, 233
    schizophrenia and, 64
    skin disorders and, 106, 112
    vaginitis and, 241
    stress incontinence, 186–87
stress management, 54–57, 64, 266–82
    see also relaxation
sugar, 31–32, 164–65, 178, 180, 253,
    312
surgery, 9, 10, 46, 137–38
sweat glands, 103–4

tampons, 243, 247
tardive dyskinesia, 63
tea, 30, 33, 58, 60, 119, 121, 185, 199, 253
tension headaches, 195–96
testes, 238–39
Tewap, 57
thalidomide, 12, 22, 254–56
tobacco, 33–34, 36
tonsillitis, 77
tonsils, 69, 77
tranquilizers, 31, 43, 46, 53–54, 112, 186,
    197, 256
transcutaneous nerve stimulators, 194, 208
travel sickness, 124
Trichomonas, 245
tryptophan, 307

ulcerative colitis, 130–31
ulcers, 35, 117
    leg, 114, 152–53
    peptic, 71, 119–23
uric acid, 216, 217
urinary incontinence, 184–88

urinary system, inflammation of (cystitis), 173, 180–84
urticaria and angioedema, 108–9

vagina:
 discharge from, 227–28, 241
 infections of, 243–46
vaginal thrush (candidiasis; yeast infection), 130, 243–45, 307–8
vaginitis and vulvovaginitis, 240–43
vasectomy, 237
vasodilators, 147
viruses, 68, 69–70, 74, 76
vitamin A, 105, 122, 253, 303
vitamin B$_6$ (pyridoxine), 51, 180, 229, 253, 257, 304
vitamin C, 76–77, 90, 162, 175, 217, 254, 304, 312
vitamin D, 253, 304
vitamin E, 90, 122, 305
vitamins, 27, 34, 253, 303–5
vomiting, *see* nausea and vomiting
vulva, 227

walking, 287–90
Wall, Patrick, 194
water drinking, 126, 128, 183, 200, 247
weight changes, menstruation and, 234
women, 77, 111, 177
 cystitis in, 180, 183
 depression in, 41, 46
 herpes in, 246–48
 infertility and, 237–40
 liver problems of, 172
 sterilization of, 237
 stress in, 271–72
 stress incontinence in, 186–87
 vaginal infections of, 240–46

yeast infection (candidiasis; vaginal thrush), 130, 243–45, 307–8
yoga, 61, 95, 276–77, 279
yogurt, 253–54

zinc, 112, 122, 160, 162, 175, 238, 305